Additional Praise for *Staying Alive*

"There is no way any of us can be 100 percent secure. However, by being properly armed with the facts and adapting even just a few of the preventive measures suggested in *Staying Alive*, we can get out of denial and fear and into healthy, appropriate action. If you want to move beyond the shock all of us experience when we hear about tragedies like Newtown, Connecticut, Aurora, Colorado, and Virginia Tech, read this book."

—Robin Hattersley Gray, Executive Editor,
Campus Safety Magazine

"I think this is an important book, easily as important as Gavin de Becker's *Gift of Fear*."

—Kenneth R. Murray, Author, *Training at the Speed of Life*

Additional Praise for the Authors

"*Innocent Targets—When Terrorism Comes to School* brings clarity and reason to a topic few people see clearly—and most people don't want to consider. Michael and Chris Dorn have done the nation an important service."

—Gavin de Becker, Captain (Ret.), LAPD,
and Best-selling Author, *The Gift of Fear*

"As one of our staff put it, learning school safety from Michael Dorn is like learning literature from William Shakespeare."

—David C. Burleson, Superintendent,
Avery County, North Carolina Schools

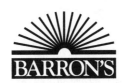

BARRON'S

STAYING ALIVE

HOW TO ACT FAST AND SURVIVE DEADLY ENCOUNTERS

MICHAEL DORN
DR. SONAYIA SHEPHERD
STEPHEN SATTERLY
CHRIS DORN

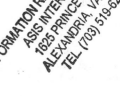

With contributions from Phuong Nguyen
and the staff of Safe Havens International

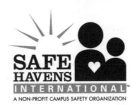

SAFE HAVENS INTERNATIONAL
A NON-PROFIT CAMPUS SAFETY ORGANIZATION

Dedication

This book is dedicated to all of those who survived the encounters described in these chapters as well as those who were not so fortunate. *Staying Alive* was written so that their losses would not be in vain.

All inquiries should be addressed to:
Barron's Educational Series, Inc.
250 Wireless Boulevard
Hauppauge, New York 11788
www.barronseduc.com

Library of Congress Catalog Card No. 2013031901
ISBN: 978-1-4380-0408-2

Library of Congress Cataloging-in-Publication Data
Dorn, Michael Stephen, 1961–
  Staying alive: how to act fast and survive deadly encounters / Michael Dorn,
Dr. Sonayia Shepherd, Stephen Satterly, Chis Dorn.
    pages cm
Includes bibliographical references and index.
ISBN 978-1-4380-0408-2
1. Survival. I. Title.
GF86.D67 2014
613.6'9—dc 23   2013031901

Printed in the United States of America
9 8 7 6 5 4 3 2 1

Contents

Contents

Acknowledgments

This book is the result of more than a year of focused writing by a five-person team with the assistance of many others. Before that year came decades of learning through the support of our friends, loved ones, clients, and colleagues. As with any book, we could not have written this alone. Fortunately, we have a great group of friends and colleagues who have helped this book become something we can be proud of.

First, we would like to thank all of the colleagues and clients that we have learned from over the years. As important as our experience as practitioners is, we are grateful for the wealth of information we have gained from each school or organization that we have assisted through our nonprofit campus safety center.

We also are blessed to have Steve Harris of CSG Literary Partners as an agent. Clearly a man of great integrity, Steve is also a tireless advocate for the authors he represents, and we are fortunate to have him as a friend and colleague.

We would also like to thank the entire Barron's team for working with us on this project and believing in our idea since its inception.

Finally, we would like to express our deepest gratitude to our families and friends who have endured countless hours of revising, opinion asking, and general advice seeking during the creation of this book.

About the Stories Used in This Book

Many of the stories in this book are based on our personal experience, the experiences of our family members, and anecdotes about our friends and colleagues. In some cases, we have changed the names or details of specific stories to protect the identities of the people involved. In four instances, we have taken some literary license with the dialogue and thought processes of people involved with the incidents who are no longer living. The details of the Enoch Brown story in the introduction, the Goleta, California, story in Chapter 5, the Red Lake Reservation School shooting story in Chapter 11, and the Iroquois Theater fire in Chapter 12 are all based on real events, and, other than the dialogue, the details of each story match the facts available about each incident.

Foreword

In September 2001, after recovering from the shock of the World Trade Center attack, virtually every American enterprise and adult began considering what steps should be taken to prevent an attack on their company, institution, or themselves personally. What had they not considered? What were the best practices and how could they be adapted locally? How would we know how well a solution would work before it was put to the ultimate test? These are fundamental questions that any risk manager would ask when assessing a potential risk of the highest severity.

My organization, Boys & Girls Clubs of America (BGCA), was no different, and we soon began receiving inquiries from many of our 1,000 local affiliate organizations, asking for examples of best practices for emergency procedures, particularly to address bomb threats and armed intruders, often referred to as active shooters. For our overall organization, no two facilities or settings are alike, and up until that time we had not considered a universal template to help all affiliates develop locally tailored plans to address a wide range of possible man-made and natural emergencies in each of the 4,000 sites they operate. Many of these sites are also shared with schools and other property owners.

As the national safety lead for our organization, I was tasked with finding a practical, actionable solution that could be infinitely adapted at the local level. What we needed did not exist because Boys & Girls Clubs are not operated exactly like schools, day care centers, Sunday schools, or most facilities where there are high concentrations of youth. No national model existed for us to readily emulate.

It was at this time that I contacted Michael Dorn, then a part of the Georgia Emergency Management Agency—Office of the

Governor (GEMA), to assist BGCA in developing emergency protocols. This began one of the most interesting and rewarding professional associations in my 35-year career with facility, safety, and security planning, and one of the most rewarding friendships of my life. As you would assume, GEMA developed the protocols for BGCA, and countless Clubs have benefited from them over the past 12 years. Michael, along with coauthors Chris Dorn (his son) and Dr. Sonayia Shepherd (who also worked on the GEMA team who assisted us), joined with school district police chief Russell Bentley to found Safe Havens International, a nonprofit center that works across the globe to make schools, places of worship, and other organizations safer.

But the true benefit came from the fact that their team not only brought a wealth of firsthand school safety and security knowledge and an understanding of security methods used around the world, but that Michael Dorn was also an alumnus—a "Club kid"—who was a member of the Boys & Girls Club of Macon, Georgia, in the 1970s. Fortunately for us, he never lost his affection for the fact that our local Clubs create safe, welcoming afterschool settings, rarely turning away a child.

I have had countless meetings and conversations with the Safe Havens team over the past 12 years, and they are truly the first people I call when I need the most realistic evaluation of a new safety or security strategy. Many of the concepts in *Staying Alive* are familiar to me as examples or solutions they have offered in years past. They bear one consistent quality: never losing sight of the ways people are likely to act or react before and after proper training.

Stories make up perhaps half of this book for good reason: they are the best way ensure the reader remembers critical lessons that are often counterinstinctive and counterintuitive. Stories also frame these life-saving lessons so that every learner easily becomes a teacher. They make us painfully aware that we owe it to the victims of past tragedies to learn from their mistakes. The authors know this and use these liberally throughout the text.

The centerpiece of this book is a simple, yet powerful concept—situational awareness. Informal situational awareness, much like the formal strategies employed in situational crime prevention, reminds us of the vital importance of using all five senses to fully understand and assess each setting in which we find ourselves. Other concepts that they will explain, such as using pattern matching, interrupting an attacker's thought process, practicing with mental simulation, using architecture and design to improve safety, verbalizing choices, and taking calculated risks all serve to train us to read the cues from the outside world and be fully prepared to survive. Under the direction of experts such as the coauthors of this book, schools have been leading the nation in the reduction of armed violence through the application of these same strategies. Sadly, these improvements largely go unnoticed or unheralded primarily because the absence of tragedy is not newsworthy.

Finally, this book answers the question "can common sense survival methods be easily taught?" The short answer is yes, but the bigger concern is whether or not people will allow themselves to be taught to survive. It is my personal wish that you will learn from the lifetimes of life-saving lessons in this book and that you will not only use them to protect yourself, but pass them along to your coworkers, friends, family, and the children who may be under your care.

Les Nichols, RA, CPP
National Vice President Child and Club Safety
Boys & Girls Clubs of America
National Headquarters
Atlanta, Georgia
October 14, 2013

INTRODUCTION

Mass casualty attacks have been a reality since the days of the one-room schoolhouse, but we can significantly reduce the chances of death not only in our schools but in other settings as well.

Arthur Dean was worried. As he walked toward home from his field-work, something nagged at him. He would feel better once he saw his boys, if he could catch them during their lunch break. He headed toward the spring near the schoolhouse to get something to drink.

As he neared the spring, he saw something lying nearby. He stopped and stood still, the sounds of the forest coming to him. Apart from the hum of insects and the chirping of birds, Arthur heard nothing. Still, he felt ill at ease. Looking toward the schoolhouse, he realized what was bothering him. The schoolhouse was silent. There was no sound of the schoolmaster's voice as he led lessons, no chorus of children's responses, no screeching of desks being moved across the wooden floorboards. Now there was only silence.

Arthur saw something lying near the spring and felt a tinge of fear. He forced himself to investigate. As he got closer, he saw that it was no inanimate object but a person—a young child. Fearful that it was one of his boys, Arthur rushed in and knelt over the child, who was covered in blood. Arthur quickly realized that this boy was not one of his sons.

The boy was moaning, repeating something over and over again. Arthur leaned in close, finally understanding what the child was whispering: "Dead, all dead!" The hair on Arthur's neck stood up.

Feeling sick to his stomach, he asked, "Boy, what's your name?"

1

At Arthur's words, the boy flinched and cried out. Laying a hand on his shoulder, Arthur spoke as gently as he could, "It's all right, boy. This is Arthur Dean. My two boys go to school with you. What's your name, son?"

As Arthur spoke, the boy seemed to calm a bit. "I-I'm A-Archie. They're all dead!"

"Archie McCullough?"

Archie started to nod, and then gasped in pain. "My head hurts!"

Arthur patted Archie on the shoulder and said, "You're safe now. Rest here, I'm going to the school."

Archie grabbed Arthur's arm and cried out, "No! They'll get you, too!"

"Who, Archie? Who will get me?" But Archie had passed out from the intense pain of his terrible wounds.

Greatly distressed, Arthur stood up and approached the one-room schoolhouse. He saw Betty Hopkins, who lived next to the school, rushing up. Pointing back, he said, "Mrs. Hopkins, Archie McCullough is over there. He's hurt, see to him. I'm going to the schoolhouse."

Arthur ran to the door of the schoolhouse and froze. The door was ajar, revealing a trail of bloody footprints. Taking a deep breath, Arthur pushed the door open and was overcome by a scene from hell.

The lifeless body of Mr. Brown, the schoolmaster, lay in front of the door and red glistened everywhere. There were ten smaller bodies covered in blood behind Mr. Brown's body. Mr. Brown and the children had been beaten to death and the tops of their heads cut off. There was a faint trail of blood from a desk to one side of the classroom. Finally, Arthur saw two recognizable shapes on the floor.

Arthur fell to his knees beside the two lifeless bodies with tears streaming down his face. Arthur's life was forever changed in the span of a few short moments (Cump, 1992).

On this dreadful day on July 26, 1764, the first known mass casualty attack at an American school took place. Our first public mass murder happened before our nation was even founded, in a one-room schoolhouse in Western Pennsylvania. With 92 percent of the occupants of the school killed, this attack is statistically the most lethal school attack to date based on mortality rates of building occupants. Even though the brutal attack at Sandy Hook Elementary school claimed more than twice as many lives, 96 percent of the building occupants survived (Sandy Hook, 2010). In fact, no attack on an educational institution in America has left such a high percentage of building occupants dead as the 1764 incident. Certainly, no mass casualty attack has been more gruesome.

While most people view school violence as a new phenomenon, this horrific event preceded more than 200 years of violence at educational facilities, shopping malls, places of work, worship, and our homes. Killers have used a wide range of weapons including guns, fire, explosives, knives, improvised weapons, biological agents, and even aircraft to murder.

Yet, during this history of violence, we have also had a magnificent history of people who have stepped up and saved lives. Sometimes this meant making the ultimate sacrifice for others. Enoch Brown and educators at Sandy Hook Elementary School died bravely in attempts to protect their students from violence. Educators in both incidents are remembered for their bravery and how they placed the safety of their students above their own (Hammel and Fleeman, 2012). Could these heroes have survived while still meeting their moral obligation to protect the innocent children under their care? Can you learn these skills to stay alive in the face of danger?

Context

These questions are not meant to judge these heroes or to judge victims of any tragedy. However, it is our responsibility to learn from past tragedies so that these deaths are not in vain. Just as the military has learned to reduce combat deaths through analysis, the rest of us can prepare for acts of violence in our daily lives. We can and must also learn from the many incidents that have been prevented.

Modern research offers powerful lessons on how we can better protect ourselves from dangerous people and situations.

It is important to remember context when considering past incidents. Without proper context, a story about interpersonal violence may as well be just another story from any war or battle. The Native Americans who carried out America's first mass casualty school attack were retaliating for an earlier attack where members of their tribe were victims of similarly shocking brutality. But even in the midst of this conflict, tribal elders were upset by the viciousness of the attack, which was made without their permission. As with many school attacks, the attack site was selected because the victims were innocent and lacked the ability to protect themselves.

Context will not make the suffering, sheer brutality, and shock of violence any less upsetting, but it will help us better understand the similarities and differences that exist between attacks at factories, office complexes, schools, shopping malls, places of worship, or any other location. Context not only is the key to understanding major acts of violence but also helps prevent its recurrence. One goal of this book is to help readers understand and plan for mass casualty acts of violence through understanding and context.

We must also keep the actual risk of being victimized in balance with other far more common causes of death. Most importantly, we must understand that we can very often protect others and ourselves from violence. Even though there are no guarantees, there are many opportunities, possibilities, and probabilities that can make it easier to stay alive if we learn and apply them.

We can also see that, contrary to popular perception, mass casualty attacks are far from a uniquely American phenomenon. As a case in point, 200 years after the first American school attack, in 1964, a former Wehrmacht soldier attacked an elementary school in Cologne, Germany, with a homemade flamethrower (Bach, 1997). The flames killed eight children and two teachers, and 22 other children were horribly burned. While the average American is painfully aware of the tragedies at Sandy Hook and Columbine, they are usually not aware that more than 200 students and staff have been shot, stabbed, or otherwise killed and injured in schools during mass casualty attacks in the People's Republic of China in recent years.

We will examine many terrible tragedies like these, but our message is one of hope, not despair. It is easy to focus on death and forget the thousands of murders that are prevented each year. This book is built on simple yet powerful concepts that can further reduce suffering. Though violent deaths will continue over time, there are many quiet successes that leave us optimistic about the future of violence prevention.

Learning to Live with a Focus on Proven Strategies

There is a natural human tendency to absorb tragedy. The 24-hour news cycle draws a lot from this primal impulse. There is certainly a need to explore these types of frightening events, but we should remember to focus on finding ways to prevent or at least survive them with a focus on real risk coupled with proven and actionable techniques.

There is no shortage of ideas for stopping violence. Installing cameras at every turn, improving mental health services, banning guns, arming schoolteachers, teaching people to attack a gunman, and a hundred other ideas are part of this discussion. At the same time, we must remember that there is no law we can pass or any single measure we can take that will eliminate such horrible events.

Through our work with Safe Havens International, our nonprofit school safety center, we see many proven approaches receive little attention while countless hours and billions of dollars are spent on unproven concepts. One primary focus of our center is to seek out validated strategies that justify the time, energy, and money that would be required to implement them. Following the same approach we use with schools, this book will focus on validated concepts that have been applied successfully to help people prevent or survive violence. The lives of human beings are too precious to take chances with speculation or ideas that may increase danger. We have seen time and time again that something that sounds good in a 30-second news story or viral video may not work so well when tested with a dangerous and determined individual.

The good news is that there are ways to reduce the chances that you or those you care about will die in a disaster. There are certain groups of people who have extensive experience in survival. Police officers, soldiers, pilots, firefighters, emergency room nurses, and others are required to operate in high-stress environments where lives are on the line every time they go to work. We can learn proven techniques from these experts in survival that can reduce the loss of life and improve the way we handle traumatic events. We will share some of this real-world experience along with research that outlines the tangible and practical steps that you can use to survive almost any situation where the opportunity to survive exists.

While we are not suggesting that you can train to the level of a Delta Force Special Operator or a SWAT commander just by reading this book, you can use some of the same techniques used by those who face life and death situations regularly to enhance your safety.

This book frequently uses shootings as examples, but it is important to note that guns are not the only weapons that have been used in mass murders. In the most fatal American K–12 school attack, the weapon was an arson fire, not a gun. The fire, which took place in 1958, was started by an elementary student and killed 95 students and staff (Boy admits, 1962; Brendtro, 2005). In this one incident, more people died than in the attacks at Columbine High School, Virginia Tech, and Sandy Hook Elementary School combined.

In 1927, a dangerously mentally ill school board member murdered more than 40 students, school employees, and bystanders with explosives (Ellsworth, 1927). As we have seen repeatedly in school attacks in the People's Republic of China, even an ordinary kitchen knife can be deadly. On the same day as the Sandy Hook Massacre, 22 students were injured with a knife in a single attack in the People's Republic of China (Sant, 2012).

The pronounced preference for many violators to use weapons other than firearms is extremely important. We desire readers to be more likely to prevent and if need be to survive any type of attack, not just those that attract intensive media coverage.

As we discuss how to react to incidents that take place despite our best attempts at preventing them, we will closely examine what you can do to protect yourself and others in the brief window of time— the first critical seconds of an emergency. In doing so, this book will show you not only how to survive deadly situations but also how you can sometimes prevent violence altogether by being observant and ready to react.

We will see that in many cases, the people who can make the most difference in a crisis are not those in a leadership or response role but everyday people who are on the front lines. The first person to spot a hazardous situation might be a custodian, an office worker, a store clerk, a teacher, a student, or a spectator at a public event. These people have an opportunity—and some might even say a responsibility—to avert tragedy. While we were writing this book, a stellar example of this took place; a school bookkeeper reacted superbly to avert an imminent tragedy at McNair Learning Academy in DeKalb County, Georgia. The bookkeeper, Antoinette Tuff, was able to persuade a heavily armed man into putting down his weapons and surrendering himself to police by relying on her own experience and having the willpower and confidence to survive. Even though at least one other staff member experienced symptoms of severe crisis stress and was unable to effectively respond to the crisis, Ms. Tuff was able to keep extraordinarily calm and collected and save lives that day (Bookkeeper talks, 2013).

As this example demonstrates, anyone could have a chance to change the outcome of a disaster. In our experience, the average person will find him- or herself in multiple situations requiring life and death decisions during a lifetime. While most of these situations will not involve a man with a rifle in a shopping mall, the outcome of each is critical. We will discuss what you can do as an individual to make your own untimely death and the sudden deaths of others less likely when the possibility for survival exists.

Parents are naturally fearful that their child may be shot and killed at a school, but it should be pointed out that a young person's chances of being killed by gunfire (or any other violent act) on school property are actually lower than their chances of being killed by lightning, a medical emergency like a bee sting, or a simple but fatal accident. In fact, violence has never been a leading cause of death in American K–12 schools. Research shows that school-related deaths typically make up less than 2 percent of all homicides among young people (Cornell, 2013).

Contrary to popular perception, the homicide rate in our schools has fallen so much over the past 30 years that tragedies like those at Sandy Hook and Virginia Tech increase the annual school homicide rate by up to 200 percent in the years in which they occur. Although it is of little consolation to those who lose a child to school violence, the fact is that fewer parents are experiencing this type of suffering because of effective improvements in school safety practices. We agree with a number of experts that there are some significant increases in the number of attempted attacks as well as in specific aspects of how they are carried out; however, comparisons of like data sets based upon per capita rates do not support the premise that school homicides have surged dramatically in recent decades. We believe the causes of the overall decrease in school homicides include improved prevention measures by schools as well as dramatic improvements in emergency medical services as has been pointed out by experts like Lt. Col. Dave Grossman.

The concepts we will explore can save lives in an active shooter attack, but these steps can also prepare you for an accidental fire, a tornado, a car wreck, a medical emergency, a lightning strike, or the most unexpected of emergencies. These same basic concepts could even be used to respond to something so outlandish as a zombie attack or a weekend in Jurassic Park. These examples are clearly fictional and may seem comical, but there are many real-life incidents that are almost stranger than fiction. Keep in mind that in early 2013 a meteor shower rained down on parts of Russia, injuring at least 1,000 people, damaging around 3,000 buildings, and requiring about 20,000 emergency responders (Russian meteor, 2013). This incident itself is reminiscent of a scene out of countless action movies with little basis in reality, but it happened. In this book, we will use many examples of bizarre yet real incidents like a student setting off a military explosive in a school by accident, a sinkhole swallowing thousands of people, and an elderly woman in leg braces nearly killing a school secretary. We will do this because research shows this can help you survive both highly unusual and more typical events.

Another common theme you will find in this book is the use of stories about people that we know, including our colleagues, friends, and family members. One of these stories illustrates the "unexpected crisis" perfectly. Deep in the jungle of the Panama Canal Zone, Private First Class (PFC) Roy Shepherd was the point man on a patrol during a training mission. As PFC Shepherd was leading the company to an assault position, he used his machete to chop low-hanging limbs to clear the path for his unit. The weather was moist and a dense fog covered much of the path.

Suddenly he felt a burning pain on his face. He soon realized that the pangs of intense pain were the stings of Africanized Honey Bees—commonly called killer bees—that descended upon him and covered much of his face, including his eyes and mouth. As he ran back to warn the company to stay out of the area, he felt his breath becoming shorter and shorter and his eyes blurred from the swelling and the bees that covered his face. He was in fact allergic to bees, so he knew that he only had a limited time to react. He quickly realized that running back to the company would put them in jeopardy because the bees were following him in attack mode. He decided to radio the other soldiers—not only to request help but also to tell the company to avoid the area. He was able to give the coordinates minutes before passing out. Shepherd woke up two days later in a hospital. The last thing that PFC Shepherd expected to encounter while fighting in the jungle was a swarm of bees, but he was able to maintain enough calm to take protective actions for his unit.

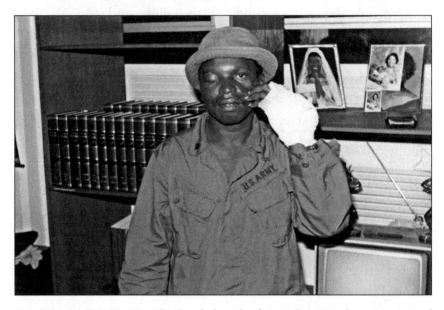

Roy Shepherd: PFC Roy Shepherd thought fast and survived an unexpected deadly encounter with killer bees in the jungles of Panama. He was able to protect himself while taking action to protect his fellow soldiers.
Photo: personal collection of Roy Shepherd

We only know of this incident because PFC Shepherd is the father of one of the coauthors. Upon reflection, the reader will likely realize that they too have family members, friends, colleagues, and acquaintances who have survived deadly encounters. Even though we often focus on the tragic events that lead to the loss of multiple lives, we must not forget what we can learn from our son-in-law who survived combat in Afghanistan, our neighbor who is a paramedic, or our uncle who escaped a deadly apartment fire many years ago.

Because our primary base of experience is heavily focused on K–12 schools, many of the examples in this book come from that setting. However, the lessons from these examples are relevant beyond schools. Most of these concepts can be applied in any setting even if they require some modification. We will also focus on cases we are personally familiar with because in these cases we have access to information that is more reliable than what would be gleaned from media accounts.

As the world's largest nongovernmental school safety center, Safe Havens International has considerable experience responding to major school tragedies and, more importantly, many situations where lives have been saved through positive practices in the school setting. Billions of dollars have been expended by state and federal government agencies to improve school safety since the 1990s, when mass casualty school attacks began to garner wide media attention. This has created a relatively new field that is growing at an even faster rate today. This experience and research has also shown us that safety is a cost-effective way to improve academic achievement over the long term.

We urge the reader to keep this in mind when we use examples from our nation's more progressive public school systems, as well as parochial, charter, and independent schools. As the reader will see, some of the nation's largest corporations could learn a great deal from school officials who have focused intently on preventing violence while providing improved service, organizational efficiency, and increased profits. The strategies employed by some of our public and independent school clients are decades ahead of what is done to protect your life when you visit some of the nation's leading big box retailers.

We will consider these challenging, complex, and difficult situations from a variety of practitioner viewpoints. The authoring team is well grounded in the fields of law enforcement, emergency management, physical security, homeland security, public health, military service, and mental health recovery. These perspectives are complimented with years of extensive research, consulting experience, postincident evaluation of seven mass casualty-shooting incidents in the United States and Canada, expert witness consultancy, as well as training and advisory work in the wake of these tragic incidents.

We have also had requests for assistance from many other sectors. Our analysts have been asked to help improve metal detection programs for the Olympic Games as well as for commercial airports in Asia. We have been asked to provide briefings for two groups of high-ranking officers from the Israeli police. We regularly train architects how to design more secure facilities and keynote homeland security conferences. The feedback on these experiences has been that the concepts covered in this book are among the most advanced available anywhere in the world. As we do with our school clients, we will focus on proven and easy-to-apply concepts. We will provide detailed background information and explanations for many concepts: however, the concepts themselves are often relatively easy to apply once you understand them.

This book also includes a series of powerful free web resources that will engage readers to see and experience important aspects of crisis prevention and response, including our Window of Life concept that can help you make decisions more effectively when you are in a life or death situation. The companion video clips and supplemental readings allow you the option to go further to prepare and empower yourself to protect human life more effectively. Readers who are interested in these topics should also consider reading the books we refer to repeatedly, like those by leaders in the field like Dr. Gary Klein, Lt. Col. Dave Grossman, Gavin de Becker, and Amanda Ripley.

One reason so many of the schools we have interacted with are so far ahead in the arena of safety, security, and emergency preparedness is because of their ability to adapt successful concepts from other sectors, like emergency medicine, commercial aviation, public safety, and the military. As the reader will see when we explore concepts like mental simulation and pattern matching and recognition, one way to improve our ability to survive is to share success strategies from one sector with others.

Throughout this book, it will be important to remember what the ultimate price for safety incidents can be. On a beautiful summer day on August 4, 1885, five thousand people gathered near Lancaster, Pennsylvania, to dedicate a memorial to Enoch Brown and his students. The granite monument is four-sided, with each side dedicated to the memory of the innocence lost. The east side of the monument lists the names of those killed, with four of the names being lost to time. The north side remembers those who donated to the park in which the monument resided. The west side gives the exact location of the remains in relation to the monument. And the south side is inscribed with a poem by Cort (1886) dedicated to the massacred:

> *The ground is holy where they fell*
> *And where their mingled ashes lie,*
> *Ye Christian people mark it well*
> *With granite column strong and high;*
>
> *And cherish well, forevermore,*
> *The storied wealth of early years,*
> *The sacred legacies of yore*
> *The toils and trials of pioneers.*

After each deadly incident large and small, we mourn our losses, ask why it happened, and then heal and get on with our lives. This cycle repeats itself, and the violence continues. We must find a way to break this cycle, to learn the skills we need to be able to prevent such violence, or at least to improve the chances of surviving it. We cannot wait for orders or for directions. No one will do this for us. We need to learn how to stay alive while remaining pragmatic yet positive and optimistic. This book is designed to take lessons from these tragedies and learn as much as we can to prevent similar events from happening in the future.

Key Points in the Introduction

- Violence is not a new phenomenon, and mass casualty attacks are far from uniquely American. Violent deaths at school make up less than 2 percent of youth homicides.

- Remember context when considering past incidents to help understand the similarities and differences that exist between attacks.
- There is a natural human tendency to absorb tragedy. Remember to focus on finding ways to prevent or survive with a focus on real risk as well as proven and actionable techniques.
- Find strategies that justify the time, energy, and money required to implement them.
- You can often prevent violence by being observant and ready to react.
- The people who can often make the most difference in a crisis are everyday people who are on the front lines. Anyone could have a chance to change the outcome of a disaster.
- Most of these concepts can be applied in any setting even if they require some modification.
- Safety is a cost-effective way to improve overall happiness, confidence, academic achievement, customer service, and profitability.

BIBLIOGRAPHY

Bach, A. (1997). Das Attentat von Koln-Volkhoven. Retrieved from *http://www.ursula-kuhr-schule.de/Chronik/Attentat/Attentat.html*

Bodeen, C. (2010). Knife-wielding man attacks 28 children at Chinese kindergarten. *The Independent.* Retrieved from *http://www.independent.co.uk/news/world/asia/knifewielding-man-attacks-28-children-at-chinese-kindergarten-1958703.html*

Bookkeeper talks about coming face-to-face with gunman. (2013, August 20). WSBTV.com. Retrieved from *http://www.ajc.com/videos/news/bookkeeper-talks-about-coming-face-to-face-with/v9ZDr/*

Boy admits fire fatal to 95. (1962, January 16). *The Miami News.* Retrieved from *http://news.google.com/newspapers?nid=71XFh8zZwT8C&-dat=19620116&printsec=frontpage&hl=en*

Brendtro, L. K. (2005). The worst school violence. *Reclaiming Children and Youth, 14*(2), 73–79.

Cornell, D. (2013) Threat assessment in Virginia schools (Presentation). Presented at the 2013 Virginia School & Campus Safety Training Forum, State D.A.R.E. and NASSLEO Conference in Hampton, Virginia on August 7.

Cump, G. L. (1992). A disquisition portraying the history relative to the Enoch Brown incident. Retrieved from *http://www.greencastlemuseum.org/index.htm*

Ellsworth, M. J. (1927). *The Bath school disaster.* Bath School Museum Committee (1991 ed.).

Ex-soldier runs amok in school. (1998). *The Standard.* Retrieved from *http://www.thestandard.com.hk/news_detail.asp?pp_cat=&art_id=42799&sid=&con_type=1&d_str=19981005&sear_year=1998*

Gado, M. (2011). *Hell comes to Bath.* TruTV.com, Turner Broadcasting. Retrieved from *http://www.trutv.com/library/crime/serial_killers/history/bath/index_1.html*

Hammel, S., and M. Fleeman. (2012, December 15). Connecticut shooting: Hero teacher died saving students. *People.* Retrieved from *http://www.people.com/people/package/article/0,,20656736_20657003,00.html*

Mahony, E,. and D. Altmari. (2012, December 15). A methodical massacre: Horror and heroics. *Hartford Courant.* Retrieved from *http://www.courant.com/news/connecticut/newtown-sandy-hook-school-shooting/hc-timeline-newtown-shooting-1216-20121215,0,5058106.story?page=1*

Man hurting 25 pupils arrested. (2004). *China View.* Retrieved from *http://news.xinhuanet.com/english/2004-09/20/content_1999428.htm*

Russian meteor blast injures at least 1,000 people, authorities say. (2013). *CNN.* Retrieved from *http://www.cnn.com/2013/02/15/world/europe/russia-meteor-shower*

Sandy Hook Elementary School overview. (2010). Connecticut Education Data and Research. Retrieved from *http://sdeportal.ct.gov/Cedar/WEB/ct_report/SnapshotGeneral.aspx*

Sant, S. V. (2012). China school knife attack leaves 23 injured. CBS News. Retrieved from *http://www.cbsnews.com/8301-202_162-57559179/china-school-knife-attack-leaves-23-injured/*

Strait, M. D. (2010). Enoch Brown: A massacre unmatched. Retrieved from *http://pabook.libraries.psu.edu/palitmap/Enoch.html*

CHAPTER ONE

ASSESSMENT AND SITUATIONAL AWARENESS

Or how to stay alert and alive.

On the afternoon of April 29, 2013, a man sat at a table in the dining room of his home while his wife and three friends sat in the adjoining living room. Abhigya, known as Abe to his friends, married his wife Erin while in college. Erin was studying to be a pharmacist, and Abe was pursuing a business finance degree. Little did the group of people in the home know that they would soon face a brutal attempt on their lives. Abe could not have dreamed how terrifying the attack would be or how his own life experience would enable him to save five lives. Abe's reaction determined the fate of everyone in the home in the most violent single minute of his life.

One of the other women present that evening was a friend named Judy. Judy and her husband were having marital issues that were interfering with her ability to study. Abe and Erin were acutely aware of this difficulty. To help Judy and her classmates concentrate while studying for finals, the group had convened for a study session. Abe was also studying, but was taking a break by browsing online videos while wearing noise-cancelling headphones. From where Abe sat, the front door was to his left, the kitchen was to his right, and the bathroom was directly in front of him.

Suddenly, the glass in the front door seemed to explode, and Judy's husband appeared in the door. Holding a hatchet in one hand and a hammer in the other, he was clearly in a violent rage. As with many acts of violence, the attack was lightning fast, brutal, and terrifying. There was no opportunity for a time out or an instant replay. The decisions that would be made in the next few seconds would determine whether five people would die a brutal and agonizing death.

The surprised group gained a few precious seconds when the attacker's hammer got caught in the door blinds. Erin took advantage of this by ushering the other women out of harm's way. One ran through the kitchen down into the basement and the other two followed Erin into the restroom and locked the door.

Abe vaguely heard the sound of breaking glass and splintering wood, but the first sign that something was horribly wrong was the sight of the four women running past him. He intuitively looked to his left and saw the angry man with the hatchet and hammer. Reacting without thinking, Abe tore off his headphones and thrust a chair at the attacker, trying to maintain distance, while screaming at him. This simple action provided another precious delay in the attacker's charge.

The aggressor knocked the chair aside, but Abe grabbed him in a headlock, taking him to the floor. During the ensuing melee, the aggressor swung at Abe with his hatchet, cutting him on his left cheek and nostril. The cut was deep enough to nick an artery, and Abe began bleeding profusely from his cheek though he did not realize it.

Abe has a black belt in *Taekwondo*, but he later recounted that in those split seconds he forgot everything he learned in his years of martial arts practice. His actions may indicate otherwise. Abe somehow managed to quickly knock the hatchet from his attacker's hand. The would-be murderer then swung the hammer, smashing Abe's forehead. Though seriously wounded, Abe was able to knock this deadly weapon out of his attacker's hand as well.

The enraged attacker fought his way on top of Abe and drew yet another hammer and began savagely beating Abe in the head with it. Though severely injured and rapidly losing blood, Abe sealed his own survival by punching his attacker in the groin. Despite attacking without remorse and having the advantage of surprise and three deadly weapons, the aggressor gave up and fled the state. He had been defeated by an unarmed but otherwise well-prepared college student.

After the attacker left, Abe went to the bathroom and the women unlocked the door. Erin began administering first aid and got a phone from the couch, where one of the women had dropped it, to call 911. While the women were trying to staunch the bleeding from Abe's cheek and other wounds, they received a chilling text message: "You are next b----es."

The assailant was found unconscious in a rest area across the state line. He had taken an entire bottle of aspirin and some Tylenol® in an attempt to take his own life. He was taken into custody and is awaiting trial at the time of this writing (Police: Man arrested, 2013).

Abe was taken to the emergency room where he received numerous stitches and more than 17 staples. Several of his teeth were chipped, too. None of the women received any physical injuries, but the emotional trauma they experienced was significant (A. Singh, personal communication, 2013).

This story is an excellent example of the importance of assessment and situational awareness. Abe and four other people are alive today because they were able to recognize the situation they were in and react rapidly enough to avert the threat. Whether you are faced with an incredibly rare situation like a shooting spree in a public place or a more typical attack like the one Abe experienced, being able to quickly assimilate information and act on it can mean the difference between life and death. In this chapter, we will explore how you can assess your surroundings to increase your chances of survival.

Situational Awareness

Two young women were sitting in a restaurant in Center City, a shopping center in Philadelphia. Maria and Cecilia were taking a break after some shopping by having some chocolate fondue. Suddenly a young male ran by. He was shirtless and seemed to be running from something.

Maria grew up in Brazil and had a broader base of experience than Cecilia. Based on that experience, she quickly picked up her phone and put it into her purse. Before she could warn Cecilia, a hand reached through the window and snatched Cecilia's phone. Not realizing the danger but reacting instinctively, Maria ran after the thief and was punched from behind. She turned to see who had punched her and saw a group of teenagers, who began taunting Maria. She went into a nearby store and called 911. Several of the teens were arrested in what was described as a "flash mob" attack (Newall, 2011).

What made Maria's reaction different than Cecilia's? Maria moved faster than her situational awareness, and as a result she placed herself in peril despite responding appropriately to the initial threat. At the same time, Celia's situational awareness evoked a different, and safer, reaction, yet she was still victimized.

According to the Marine Corps, situational awareness is the knowledge and understanding of the current situation that promotes a timely, relevant, and accurate assessment of situations within your area in order to facilitate decision making (Department of the Navy, 2011). As both an informational perspective and a skill set, situational awareness fosters an ability to determine the context and relevance of events that are rapidly unfolding. Situational awareness is a learned skill that can help us prevent violence or reduce the damage from violence we cannot prevent.

Situational awareness means collecting information about your surroundings so you can respond according to what is happening at any given moment. It starts when we enter any area for the first time and ends with our last visit. It is what we do as part of our daily routine and is an invaluable basic survival trait. When we take the time to program our brain properly, it can be our most powerful survival tool.

When we drive a car, our brain observes the activity around us, making hundreds of calculations, most of which we are not even aware of as we perform them. We must continuously assess speed, distance, and probabilities. These skills do not just materialize automatically. We make a deliberate effort to train ourselves to drive, and with experience these skills become second nature. And, usually, the more we drive, the better we get, since we expand our base of knowledge and experience. Once we learn how to drive and feel comfortable with the process, we often perform tasks related to driving without even thinking. How many times have you driven to or from work without consciously thinking about what you were doing? And how many times have you taken a wrong turn because you needed to deviate from your normal route to run an errand?

Situational awareness is a continual assessment process (Sherwood, 2009). For example, police officers are trained to automatically identify, scan, and remain aware of people's hands when they interact with the public. Most weapons require the use of our hands, so learning to scan people's hands, especially when someone is angry or exhibiting other warning signs, is an excellent habit. Each of us encounters angry or potentially dangerous people from time to time. Though we often fail to realize it, many of us come into contact with armed individuals from time to time. Even though many of these people never use these weapons, knowing that a person is armed could change the way we handle many common situations. It can also save our lives.

To develop situational awareness, you must use all of the senses available to you, including sight, smell, sound, taste, and touch. Barring any physical challenges we may face, we have been collecting information with these senses all our lives. During a crisis, these senses can save our lives. This happens so often that we sometimes take it for granted. Try to recall how many times you have barely averted being hit by a vehicle while walking, riding a bicycle, or driving a car? Our senses can be used individually or, as they often are, in concert with one another.

Another component of situational awareness is recognizing where you are. This is more than just knowing *where* you are, but knowing this in relation to the larger world around you. Paying attention to available exit routes, safe locations, potential obstacles, and other factors provides you with options and alternatives in an emergency. This information can significantly increase your odds of survival. For example, if your office were filled with smoke, would you remember which direction you need to go to get out of danger, keeping in mind that you might be crawling on your hands and knees because of the smoke. Or if you are walking through an office building and a gunman or a dangerously mentally ill woman with a butcher knife approached you, would you intuitively know to select a viable path to safety? In our world today, it is easy to get distracted by a sensory overload and forget where we are.

Everyone naturally conducts these informal assessments to one degree or another. It is simply a matter of learning how to expand that ability to include today's broader range of environmental and situational risks. Research on how college students rate their professors found that students could accurately judge a professor's quality with only two seconds of observing his or her teaching style (Gladwell, 2005). As individuals, we can develop these skills along with our natural survival instincts (i.e., our ability to make informal assessments) for today's risks. We are descendants of people who had to evade predators and compete for food, water, and shelter. Today we have to contend with people who may shoot us, stab us, beat us with a baseball bat, or, more commonly, slam into our car as they text while driving.

If you are a parent, you may have had discussions with your child about the differences between hearing and listening. Too often, our body senses something dangerous, but denial or ignorance causes us to not pay attention to our own observations. Our senses are constantly working and gathering data, and our task is to learn to effectively harness the power of these senses even when we are focused on other things. In the story of Maria and Cecilia, both saw the youth running down the road. Maria reacted differently than Cecilia, and she was able to secure her phone. Later you will learn why Maria was still unable to detect the crowd of teens that would assault her as she ran out the door.

Another good way to describe situational awareness is the concept of an OODA loop. OODA stands for Observe, Orient, Decide, and Act. It was developed by Colonel John Boyd of the U.S. Air Force as a means of determining why some fighter pilots are better than others. It is now used in litigation, business, and other commercial enterprises, as well as in military strategy, law enforcement, and anything else that involves potential conflict between one or more parties (Boyd, 1976). Interpersonal conflict can thus be seen as a series of interlocking OODA loops. If you can find a way to interrupt your opponent's OODA loops or getting inside their OODA loops, then you can gain the upper hand.

Let us return to the situation faced by Abe and Erin. The attacker had a plan when he entered Abe and Erin's house. He was going to kill his wife Judy. When he forced his way into the house, the attacker began a new OODA loop. He observed the four women, one of them his wife, running into another room. He also observed Abe, who is a fairly large man, getting up and taking off his headphones. His orientation toward his wife was interrupted by Abe's presence.

Abe, on the other hand, observed the women running into the bathroom and kitchen and then saw the attacker with weapons. He oriented to the threat and quickly placed a chair in front of the aggressor. After being slashed in the face, Abe observed the chair being thrown out of the way. He reoriented to the hatchet and knocked it away. He performed similar loops for the attacks with each of the hammers. He was then able to get inside the attacker's OODA loop and punch him in the groin, effectively ending the attack. The attacker was oriented toward killing his wife, but Abe's actions kept interfering with both his orientation toward his wife and the secondary orientation of getting Abe out of the way. This allowed Abe to disrupt what the attacker wanted to do and gave Abe more time to react. When analyzing an attempted violent crime, the OODA loop can help you understand how it happened and can provide you with valuable insights for future reference.

Situational awareness can be an informal process that integrates into our everyday life, or it can be a more formal process we engage in with others. It can be as simple as learning pathways, potential obstacles, available resources, and shelter locations. We are asked to enhance our situational awareness each time we fly on commercial aircraft by the phrase "Locate the nearest emergency exit—the nearest exit may be behind you."

While working with the Yorktown Central School District in New York, coauthor Michael Dorn got to know Assistant Superintendent Tom Cole. His father, Thomas Cole, was the chief of police in Bronxville, New York. Tom recounted a story from his childhood of how he and his brother and sisters learned a survival technique from their father. He would make them cover their eyes when they were in a restaurant and ask them to quickly identify various emergency escape routes. To this day, Mr. Cole automatically notes emergency exits and other avenues of escape when he enters a building.

Using age-appropriate examples and language, this simple technique can help children and adults learn how to live if they encounter a violent aggressor, a fire, or any other type of emergency that requires immediate evacuation. As we will reiterate, 5 to 30 seconds can, and often does, mean the difference between life and death in an emergency. Our ability to recognize and respond to danger in the first precious seconds of an emergency is one of the most critical life-saving concepts known to mankind. Whether you fly a fighter aircraft with extensive computer warning systems or are a pedestrian walking down the street, your ability to quickly assess a situation and recognize and react to danger may determine whether you and other people live or die.

In a crisis, we must be prepared to quickly make critical decisions based on the often limited and rapidly changing information we have available at any given moment. Increasing the amount or accuracy of the information available to us improves our ability to make life-saving decisions quickly and correctly. Taking time to gather information can and often does lead to the right decision. Unfortunately, taking too much time to gather information can also result in death or serious injuries because our reactions are too slow to be effective. Learning and developing situational awareness skills helps you react faster in crisis situations.

Conclusion

Abe's self-defense response seemed instinctive. However, the research of Dr. Gary Klein shows that our instinctive reactions are based on our brain's amazing ability to draw on the experiences gained over our lifetimes (Klein, 2004). Abe's martial arts training gave him the skills he needed to repeatedly disarm his opponent. His training also provided him with the means to make these assessments quickly and make decisions based on that information. By practicing and developing these skills as simple habits, you can enhance your situational awareness over time with little disruption to your daily life.

We hope and pray that you never have to face anything resembling the terror that Abe and Erin felt when a violent man burst through their front door. But hoping will not make evil people go away. The things Abe and Erin did *before* the attack allowed them to stay alive. In just a few seconds, they simplified their choices by prioritizing their goals, observed the aggressor's actions, oriented to their top priority, decided what to do, and acted. They did so effectively and survived their ordeal.

You may or may not have the inherent instincts shown by Abe and Erin. You may or may not possess the close combat skills demonstrated by Abe. But regular practice, simple assessment skills, and prioritization can often help you avoid getting into these situations at all. If an attack does occur, understanding how to interrupt an aggressor's OODA loop can help you come out on top.

While mass shootings and terrorist bombings dominate media coverage, you are more likely to face an act of interpersonal aggression like the one Erin and Abe experienced (de Becker, 2002). There are literally tens of thousands of such attacks every year. This makes it important to understand that there are numerous ways in which people may have to face violence. Rape/sexual assault, domestic violence, violent crime, and armed robbery are among the many types of violence that happen every day. Looking at the statistics, we know that although Abe and Erin's ordeal was not chronicled by news networks, it is much more typical of the types of events that happen with the most frequency. Abe and Erin's story should assist you in recognizing, preventing, and facing not only the types of violence that dominate the news but everyday acts, too. These lessons should also enhance your ability to respond to almost any life-threatening, fast-breaking emergency like a tornado, a fire, a car accident, or an extremely unlikely attack by a Great White Shark.

It should be pointed out that the people in Abe and Erin's story live in a quiet Midwestern town that has a low rate of violent crime. The community has an excellent, well-trained police force that helps to keep violence relatively rare. Driving through these neighborhoods, one might describe them as idyllic. Yet, violence suddenly came into this peaceful town. A slight change in fortunes may have seen the headline "Brutal slaying of four" in a town where people say, "It wouldn't happen here." This attack should be a wake-up call to college students, schoolteachers, factory workers, mechanics, receptionists, chief executive officers, and stay-at-home parents. The incident reminds us that there is some risk of violence anywhere in the world.

Key Points in Chapter One

- The ability to quickly assimilate and act on information can mean the difference between life and death.
- A continual assessment process, situational awareness is a learned skill that can help prevent violence or reduce the damage from violence we cannot prevent.
- A window of time—sometimes as short as 5 to 10 seconds—can mean the difference between life and death in an emergency. The ability to recognize and respond to danger in the first seconds

of an emergency is one of the most critical life-saving concepts known to mankind.

- Learning and developing situational awareness skills helps to react faster in crisis situations. Taking too much time to gather information can result in death or serious injuries.
- Instinctive reactions are based on the brain's ability to draw on the experiences gained over our lifetimes.
- Practice, simple assessment skills, and prioritization can help you avoid getting into these situations at all.
- Understanding how to interrupt an aggressor's OODA loop can help you to survive an attack.

For more about Abe and Erin's story, visit *www.SafeHavens International.org.*

BIBLIOGRAPHY

de Becker, G. (2002). *Fear Less: Real Truth About Risk, Safety, and Security in a Time of Terrorism.* Boston: Little, Brown and Company.

Boyd, J. R. (1976). *Destruction and creation.* Retrieved from *http://www.goalsys. com/books/documents/DESTRUCTION_AND_CREATION.pdf*

Department of the Navy, U.S. Marine Corps. (2011). *Marine Corps supplement to the Department of Defense dictionary of military and associated terms.* Retrieved from *http://www.marines.mil/Portals/59/Publications/MCRP%20 5-12C%20Marine%20Corps%20Supplement%20to%20the%20DoD%20 Dictionary%20of%20Military%20and%20Associated%20terms.pdf*

Gladwell, M. (2005). *Blink: The power of thinking without thinking.* New York: Back Bay Books.

Klein, G. (2004). *The power of intuition: How to use your gut feelings to make decisions at work*: New York: Crown Business.

Newall, M. (2011). Teens in a mob assault and rob Center City patrons. *Philadelphia Inquirer.* Retrieved from *http://articles.philly.com/2011-06-29/ news/29717406_1_maria-teens-mob-assaultKnight*

Police: Man arrested on attempted murder charges after hatchet attack. (2013). *Crimetracker.* Retrieved from fox59.com website: *http://fox59.com/2013/05/ 02/police-man-arrested-on-attempted-murder-charges-after-hatchet-attack/ #axzz2Up2TUHD2*

Sherwood, B. (2009). *The survivors club: The secrets and science that could save your life.* New York: Grand Central Publishing.

CHAPTER TWO

"PEOPLE DETECTORS"— USING PATTERN MATCHING AND RECOGNITION TO DETECT DANGER

How your brain can detect the subtle but critical signs of danger.

Three young men approached the campus of McEvoy Middle School and waited a short distance away. Though still young, they had hard hearts and evil intent. They had come prepared to kill, and their target was just a boy. They did not care that he was just a child or that the school was a place where children should be safe and unafraid. They were gang members, intent on making a statement. The boy belonged to a gang that had shot one of their members, and this must be avenged. The boy had to pay, and he had to pay with his life.

The gang members wanted to avoid the tight security at the school, so they waited on an adjacent street. They chose it because the school bus would turn onto it as it left the safe haven of the campus. They planned to intercept the bus and kill the young boy without interference. What these men had not counted on was Officer Kenneth Bronson. They were also unaware of this officer's particular skills—specifically, a skill set now called *pattern matching and recognition*. Officer Bronson's experience allowed him to detect, identify, and respond to subtle behavioral cues that told him the young men were up to no good. He had established an understanding of the normal behavior patterns in the community, and he recognized something different that day. Most importantly, he took action. Because of Officer Bronson's skill at noticing minor details on crowded school campuses at peak times of the day, the boy would safely return to his parents.

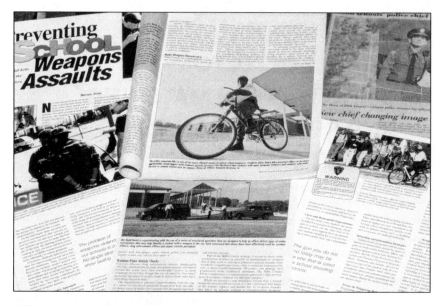

Officer Bronson: The amazing exploits of Officer Bronson and his fellow officers in the Bibb County Schools Police Department were featured in hundreds of national news stories and magazine articles.
Photo: Rachel Wilson, articles courtesy of Police Magazine *and* School Planning & Management.

The simple but powerful concepts that Officer Bronson used can be applied by anyone in any setting to make people safer. The field of nursing first formally identified the concept of pattern matching and recognition with great success. Researchers also now know how people like Officer Bronson are able to notice seemingly innocuous behaviors at such a great distance. The human brain has the potential to detect and react to some types of danger more rapidly and more accurately than a computer (Klein, 1998). More importantly, we will see how you can learn and apply this powerful and proven concept to take charge of your own personal safety.

Pattern Matching and Recognition

The concept of pattern matching and recognition, also referred to as *pattern matching,* was first formally developed in cardiac care units in the United Kingdom. In his book *Know What You Don't*

Know—How Great Leaders Prevent Problems Before They Happen,
Dr. Michael Roberto, a trustee professor of management at Bryant
University, explains how these cardiac units began offering additional training for nurses—a level of training that had previously
been provided only to doctors. In many situations, nurses spend
more time with patients and can therefore sometimes have a greater
awareness of any changes to the patient's physical condition than a
doctor. Because of this, the nurses were given training on how to
spot indications of a second or subsequent heart attack for the high-
risk patients in cardiac units.

The nurses quickly became more effective at summoning rapid
response teams (some people call them "crash carts" or "code blue"
teams) who could quickly evaluate the situation and take the actions
necessary to save a patient's life. Though costly, these rapid response
teams perform highly effective medical tests and procedures to stop
an impending heart attack. This became known as "pattern matching" since it relied heavily on the ability of nurses to look for specific
patterns in EKG readouts as indicators of an impending emergency.
The idea of providing additional pattern-matching training for
nurses proved to be extremely effective and quickly spread to hospitals around the world (Roberto, 2009).

In Australia, another group of innovative medical professionals
decided to add one seemingly minor adjustment when they implemented pattern matching. One simple modification has since saved
the lives of countless people. Just like the nurses in England, these
nurses were trained on how to watch for tangible indicators, like
changes in a patient's heartbeat patterns. The chance came when
they were given the additional imperative that they were empowered, and expected, to activate a rapid response team whenever they
saw anything outside the norm of behaviors they had come to expect
from patients with similar medical conditions. In other words, they
were told to look for behaviors that seemed odd or out of place,
much like the "gut feeling" that Officer Bronson listened to when
he noticed something minor but out of the ordinary. This approach

combined two areas of expertise: the tangible and often measurable physical symptoms as well as the nurses' personal work experience. Law enforcement officers, soldiers, and many others whose job is to protect us now use this same basic concept.

Gavin de Becker has thoughtfully explained this same type of observation. De Becker is considered to be among the world's top experts on the signs and types of violent behavior. In his superb book *The Gift of Fear and Other Survival Signals That Protect Us from Violence*, de Becker provides excellent illustrations of how our brains can detect danger if we do not ignore what we see and hear (de Becker, 1997). De Becker provides specific "danger signals" that we can look for, but also emphasizes the power of the human brain to notice abnormal patterns of behavior.

By applying pattern matching, you are more likely to be alerted to specific details more quickly. To apply these concepts, you must learn to trust yourself, trust your work experience, and, most importantly, trust your life experience. Your brain is a highly developed protective system, as long as you do not shut it off.

In an interview for our training video series *The First 30 Seconds*, Lt. Col. Grossman says, "the human brain is the most powerful survival mechanism known to man" (Dorn, 2012). Grossman is a retired army ranger and former psychology instructor at West Point who has conducted extensive research on the human mind in a state of crisis, leading to his two excellent books—*On Killing* and *On Combat*. According to Grossman, de Becker, Roberto, and Klein, what we often credit to "intuition" is actually our brain matching sensory observations with our base of experience using swift mental calculations.

In other words, intuition is often based on pattern matching and recognition. These patterns may involve a simple difference in tone of voice, or the way a person is standing, walking, or talking. While we can easily understand the veteran cop on the beat noticing that something does not look quite right, we often fail to take into account that all people have life experience and a brain that can detect words and actions that are incongruent for the context. Your ability to spot patterns should be based on your life experiences. These experiences uniquely qualify your brain to notice subtle cues for the places you frequent, like your place of work, worship, recreation, or residence.

The Bureau of Alcohol, Tobacco, Firearms, and Explosives (BATFE) employs some of America's top bomb experts. The BATFE advises that ordinary people are often more capable of detecting an explosive device in a familiar setting than a trained law enforcement officer responding to a bomb threat. This is because a skilled bomber can make a bomb look like almost anything or place it in any container like a box, book bag, purse, or briefcase. Employees who are taught basic concepts of visually scanning their work areas are more likely to detect a device (U.S. Department of Homeland Security, 2013). This is one example of an application of pattern matching. A dangerous person might not draw the attention of a police officer driving past a city park across the street from your home, but you might be able to notice that one person in the area does not act like the people who typically frequent the park. This in turn may make it easier for you than the well-trained police officer to spot a child molester or burglar in your neighborhood. The ability of your brain to detect danger applies to muggers, rapists, burglars, people who are about to open fire in a public place, and terrorists. No matter how hard they try, none of these individuals will act exactly the same way as a harmless person.

Retail businesses can also benefit from pattern matching. One day, two employees of a sporting goods store noticed that a customer was acting suspiciously as he approached their front entrance. They were so concerned with his behavior that one of them retrieved a semiautomatic pistol, holding the gun out of sight under the counter after loading a round into the chamber just as the man entered the store. The man apparently recognized the sound of the gun being loaded and nervously commented that he did not realize the store sold firearms. After mentioning that he thought the store sold athletic equipment, he rapidly departed.

Wondering if they had overreacted, the employees began to discuss why the man's behavior had alarmed them. The man was wearing a long coat, even though it was a very hot day. He had also nervously looked around just before entering the store, perhaps scanning for witnesses. Finally, they had noticed that his right arm was bent at an awkward angle while he was in the store. Although they had not been trained to look for these specific cues, they had reacted to them because they trusted their instincts.

The employee who pulled and loaded a handgun did not point the weapon at the man, but he readied himself to do so. Law enforcement officers later told them that a man closely matching the same description had robbed a number of stores in the neighborhood. The man apparently kept a sawed off shotgun in his coat sleeve, which explained the odd position of his arm that had drawn their attention. Their fast reaction almost certainly averted an armed robbery and perhaps an even more serious outcome. Prior to analyzing what had caused them to react, the employees only knew that customers did not act that way.

The Applications

Since first being used by nurses in the cardiac unit, the concept of pattern matching and recognition has spread to many other fields. If you are taken hostage, and a SWAT team performs a tactical rescue, the first officers through the door will probably use pattern matching and recognition to quickly identify anyone in the room who may be armed. The brave men of SEAL Team Six likely used pattern matching and recognition at a nonstop pace to minimize the loss of life in the raid on the Bin Laden compound while also rapidly determining which of the many people in the compound posed a threat.

In these situations, pattern matching helps direct their attention to the dangerous people in the room so they can be ready to shoot quickly, and only shoot at the right people, if need be. It will also help them react more quickly even if there are 50 or more people to quickly assess. To avoid the inappropriate use of lethal force, police officers often need to be capable of quickly evaluating a situation and deciding how to respond. Pattern matching and recognition makes it possible for hostages as well as those who put their lives on the line to protect themselves and return safely to their families each day.

To understand this aspect of pattern matching more fully, let us return to the story of Officer Bronson. This officer was a handpicked member of the elite Special Operations Unit in the Bibb County School System Police Department. Led by a former U.S. Navy SEAL, the unit was made up of three highly motivated and diverse officers. At the time, this unit was part of one of the nation's most highly trained and well-equipped law enforcement agencies. Each officer in the department received an average of six weeks of police academy training every year and fired 3,000 rounds of ammunition during range training. This was far more training than provided to most local, state, or federal law enforcement agencies at the time.

Using concepts learned from across the nation as well as from the Israeli police and military units, these dedicated men and women were on the cutting edge of the prevention of school shootings, helping to develop and popularize many techniques that have now been used to stop countless planned school shootings around the country. For example, officers in the department used a concept known as visual weapons screening to avert several shooting incidents. This skill set allows a person to spot the specific physical behaviors that can indicate a person is carrying a weapon. The officers in Bibb County used these and other techniques to prevent school shootings years before the Columbine High School attack. Officer Bronson was especially well trained, equipped, highly motivated, and particularly skilled in applying pattern matching. He also had an uncanny ability to apply visual weapons screening. This enabled him to stop these dangerous and highly determined men on that school day.

Just as importantly, Officer Bronson worked in a school system that had created a culture that not only allowed but also expected him to act when he noticed subtle differences in human behavior. Sitting atop a police mountain bicycle more than three football field lengths away, Officer Bronson noticed something. What he noticed was not alarming at first, and it was not something that would catch the eye of most people. But what he saw made him immensely curious; though a minor detail, it was something he had never seen before. It compelled him to quickly ride over to the bus pickup area to satisfy that curiosity. He wanted to know why the students lined up at the school bus were not boarding the bus.

For the average person, the empowerment required to use and act upon observable patterns of human behavior is internal. Your fear of being perceived as "crying wolf" can be the biggest roadblock to detecting and reacting to danger. Observing the patterns is not enough. To make a difference, you have to act promptly when you detect an unusual pattern.

When Officer Bronson approached the bus, he noticed the three young men standing across the street from the school. Officer Bronson asked the students what was wrong. They quickly explained that the three men were gang members and that they were mad at one of the students who rode the bus. They were afraid the men might be planning to shoot at the boy as the bus departed. Even middle school kids can, and often do, use pattern matching and recognition.

Officer Bronson ordered the students to safety and reflexively called for backup. He then approached the three men with his hand on his pistol. He ordered them to keep their hands in plain sight and walked toward them. As he neared the opposite side of the two-lane street, he applied specific training on visual weapons screening. Because of this formal training, Officer Bronson was particularly skilled at recognizing physical indicators like the outline of what turned out to be a very small, but potentially lethal, .25 caliber semiautomatic pistol in the right front pocket of one of the outlaws. Officer Bronson quickly used his service pistol to successfully avert "yet another planned school shooting" without firing a shot.

Pattern matching drew Officer Bronson to the scene from 300 yards away. His rapport with students and the reputation of the school police department created a situation where the students felt comfortable sharing their fears. His training on specific cues then enabled him to correctly determine that one of the men was indeed armed. His immediate reaction of drawing his service pistol occurred fast enough to prevent the gang members from opening fire.

In his groundbreaking research on decision making, Klein found that veteran firefighters are usually quickly able to spot and identify dangerous situations they have never encountered before. The experience of working hundreds and even thousands of fires enabled veteran fire commanders to detect subtle differences in fires that allowed them to correctly identify these new dangerous situations (Klein, 1998). In the same manner, a factory worker is often well prepared to notice a coworker who is preparing to carry out an attack at the job site—if the worker does not ignore what he or she sees or hears.

This life-saving concept has averted the deaths of hospital patients, dignitaries, police officers, soldiers, and many others where it has been put into use. Officer Bronson used it to prevent the death of the young boy nearly two decades ago. People have also used these skill sets to prevent death in many other settings. It is one of the best opportunities to make our schools, movie theaters, offices, places of worship, and homes much safer.

Another great thing about pattern matching is that it can make schools more effective places of learning, businesses more profitable, parents more connected to their children, workplaces more pleasant, and places of worship even more tightly knit. This is because it forces us to become more aware of the needs of others. This approach also helps us avert issues with more common concerns like school bullying, teen substance abuse, sexual harassment in the workplace, employee theft, fraud, and a wide range of other destructive behaviors.

The Power of Experience and Training

Like Officer Bronson, some people are naturally gifted at using pattern matching without any formal training. Glenn Rotkovich, the owner of the Lead Valley Gun Range, told reporters that he received an application from the alleged shooter in the Aurora Theater mass shooting about a month before the attack. When he called the man's apartment to follow up on the application, he heard a strange voice message.

"His answering machine message was incoherent, just bizarre, really bizarre—slurring words, but he didn't sound drunk, just strange—I could make out 'James' somewhere in it," said Mr. Rotkovich (Winter, 2012). "In hindsight, looking back—and if I'd seen the movies—maybe I'd say it was like the Joker—I would have gotten the Joker out of it," he said. "It was like somebody was trying to be as weird as possible" (Winter, 2012). The application also had some strange signals that struck the range owner further. Mr. Rotkovich did not ignore his intuition and instructed all of his employees not to allow Holmes to join the range until he personally had a chance to interview him. He noticed the differences in Holmes's behavior in contrast to the many other people who had inquired about the range over the years.

While handling a call at a Georgia department store in the mid 1970s, responding police officers learned that an adult male had been shoplifting with the help of a young child who was clearly too young to understand what he was doing. The man had been giving the boy items to place in a bag and then walked out of the store, with the boy carrying the bag. Two store security officers had been watching this activity and challenged the man as soon as he left the store. The man ran, leaving the child and the stolen goods.

After the security officers described the man, one of the veteran officers immediately noticed the suspect standing across a four lane roadway about 250 yards away and wearing a different color shirt and pants. He told other officers not to look, since they would alert the suspect. Naturally, everyone in the group immediately looked in the man's direction. The suspect fled once again but was apprehended after a lengthy chase.

Afterward, a colleague asked the officer how he had spotted the man. Everyone was surprised that this officer had been able to identify a suspect who did not fit the description provided, who was standing so far away, and who was shielded by four lanes of heavy traffic and standing among hundreds of pedestrians in the area. The officer responded that the man simply did not act like any of the hundreds of other people around. He then realized that other than the color of the clothing, the man fit the general description in terms of height and weight. More importantly, the man appeared to be very nervous, and his gaze was fixated on the scene of the investigation. The man had gone home, changed clothing, and returned to the area.

Like Officer Bronson, this officer was not provided with any formal training in pattern matching. Through his experience responding to thousands of calls over the years, he learned to trust his instincts. Like Officer Bronson, this officer was also an astute observer of human behavior, and his colleagues just assumed it was some kind of sixth sense. Similarly, firefighters, along with experts in other fields Dr. Klein has studied, develop this type of response ability through thousands of hours of experience. A clerk in a home improvement store can also spot the customer who does not act like thousands of others because she has entered the store to kill her ex-husband who works there.

Pattern matching also requires training on how to pay attention to the subtle differences in human behaviors that can indicate danger rather than ignoring them, as many people do by default. People can be trained to look for these differences, which are not always blatant and obvious but can be easily noticed by people who have given themselves permission to observe and act. Today, police officers, soldiers, teachers, school bus drivers, custodians, secretaries, office managers, and many others are being provided with formal training that can help them learn to spot these patterns when they have not developed these skills on their own just as Officer Bronson did. Certain people in an organization can be in a very good position to use pattern matching. Receptionists, secretaries, custodians, human resources personnel, maintenance personnel, and parking attendants are among the types of people who are often in an excellent position to spot and react to danger. For example, pattern matching can help a receptionist detect signs of danger when screening visitors in person or over an intercom system. As Mr. Rotkovich demonstrated, patterns of concern can be heard as well as seen.

Explaining the concept and telling people to pay attention to gut feelings is a big step in unleashing the power of employees in any organization or members of your own family. Telling people not to ignore an uneasy feeling and to ask themselves why they are uncomfortable about someone can lead to the recognition of more overt behaviors. Each of us has certain areas of interest and focus that allow us a unique perspective and ability to detect danger.

It is also important to understand that criminals often use these same methods to detect easy victims. For example, pickpockets and robbers have for decades targeted tourists in New York City by spotting people whose actions are different from those of local residents, such as constantly looking up at the city's many tall buildings. Criminals know that tourists are less likely to detect them as quickly and are not likely to return to the city to testify against them if they are caught.

This can be especially important when traveling abroad because tourists are often favorite targets of criminals in other countries for the same reasons. Trying to blend in can reduce your risks when you travel. While this may not be as easy to do in some places, there are many instances where it is possible. Even the simple act of demonstrating a sense of personal awareness can mitigate the vulnerability of your position.

Coauthor Chris Dorn has used the concepts of visual screening to give the impression that he is armed when walking in foreign countries and even high-crime areas in the United States. When he travels to places like Bolivia and Vietnam, it is obvious that he is not a local resident, but he has successfully used body language cues to signal to potential pickpockets and thieves that he is not an easy target. This is particularly helpful in Bolivia, where criminals sometimes use fake police cars and police stations to extort money from foreigners.

These skills are just as critical in seemingly safe locations like tourist destinations and theme parks. Coauthors Michael Dorn and

Chris Dorn were presenting at a large police convention at an internationally renowned resort and theme park when a rash of break-ins were reported in the conference center parking deck. The thieves had focused on breaking into police vehicles because of the false sense of security of conference participants and the knowledge that valuable items like guns and computers might be stored in these vehicles.

Pattern matching helps to support and reinforce other types of training. For example, teachers may notice the indications of bullying more quickly or help prevent a child from dropping out of school through its use. Parents may spot a son or daughter who is at risk for suicide or to detect a sexual predator who is "grooming" a child for abuse. Business owners can use pattern matching to avoid hiring or investment mistakes. In schools, pattern matching can prevent a school shooting, and it can help raise test scores. Because it improves connectivity between people, pattern matching can improve interactions and customer service. If you have received some form of training on how to spot specific behaviors that can be indicators of danger, pattern matching can enhance these skills.

Pattern matching can also help to reduce the chances that unintentional racial profiling will occur. This is because pattern matching relies on the behaviors rather than the physical characteristics of people. As Gladwell points out in his book *Blink,* there is extensive evidence that people are often more suspicious of certain ethnic minorities such as African Americans, even if they are of the same race (Gladwell, 2005). While pattern matching will not help reduce any intentional use of racial profiling, it is our experience that people who use pattern matching tend to focus on race less because they are looking for behavioral indicators rather than physical characteristics.

Better Safe Than Sorry

It is important to explain that the nurses who first used these concepts were assured they would not be chastised for false alarms. This is because the effective use of pattern matching requires permission (both from others as well as yourself) to be less than 100 percent accurate in noting and reacting to unusual patterns of behavior. This level of empowerment allowed nurses to trust their own judgment and intuition. It is better to be embarrassed than to miss the chance to prevent death or injury. The additional training, combined with the simple act of empowering the nurses to unleash the incredible power of their brains, reduced mortality in cardiac units by as much as 50 percent (Roberto, 2009). This is a pretty significant improvement considering it means half as many people died in these units.

This fear of being embarrassed if we are wrong (and embarrassing those whose actions we question) can be a powerful impediment to survival. For example, in a 1956 research study by the U.S. Air Force, a variety of factors were found to explain why fighter pilots often failed to eject when their planes were about to crash. While there were some impediments to safe ejection caused by systems that were too complex, a major factor was determined to be the failure of pilots to eject because they were too concerned with their reputation among their supervisors and peers if they ejected. For example, researchers learned from pilots who had successfully ejected that they had often delayed the decision to eject when the need to eject was clear-cut. By redesigning aircraft ejection systems and training programs, the Air Force was able to reduce the number of pilots killed in these types of accidents. Instilling permission to eject from an aircraft when it is appropriate was a major component (Beer et al., 1961). When even highly trained fighter pilots can die because of peer pressure, imagine how much of a barrier this can be to the average person.

Just as fighter pilots and nurses are trained to focus on what needs to be done and ignore the fear of how others might perceive their actions, you must mentally prepare yourself to listen to your brain to spot danger and take immediate action. This can be much harder than it sounds. We spend our entire lives being second-guessed and criticized in work and social settings. We are sometimes so concerned about what other people think of us that we can find ourselves doing things that are truly not logical. Our concern for public perception can quickly get out of balance. It can, and sometimes does, result in our failure to recognize danger and react to it fast enough.

People Detectors

Bill Modzeleski, who served for many years as the point man for school safety for the U.S. Department of Education, was once asked what he thought about using metal detectors to prevent school shootings. His response to the question was both revealing and in line with what research, experience, and postshooting forensic evaluation tells us. Modzeleski replied that although metal detectors are appropriate for some schools, every school needs more effective "people detectors."

Like the authors, Modzeleski felt that school staff who are properly trained, connected, and sensitive to the students they serve are in a good position to prevent school violence. Officer Bronson is a prime example of an effective people detector. Taking it to a broader environment, people detectors can help prevent violence from happening to themselves and other people in any setting.

Conclusion

Pattern matching is just one example of the set of tools that can help to create more effective people detectors in our schools, our businesses, our places of worship, and our homes. From cardiac care units, to SWAT teams, to bank staff, school employees, and those at our places of worship, pattern matching is successfully being used on a daily basis to avert violence, to prevent suicides, and to keep at-risk youth in school. There is usually less media attention given to a tragedy that is prevented, but these successes are incredibly important. A proven, practical, and powerful tool, pattern matching can make you and those you care about much safer from dangerous individuals while improving your connection with those around you.

Key Points in Chapter Two

- The human brain can detect and react to some types of danger more rapidly and accurately than a computer.
- You are more likely to be alerted to specific signs of danger more quickly by applying pattern matching and recognition.
- If you do not ignore what you see and hear, your brain can detect danger.
- Your ability to spot patterns should be based on your life experiences.
- Intuition is often based on pattern matching and recognition and helps to direct attention to dangerous people or situations.
- Visual weapons screening is a skill set that allows someone to spot the specific physical behaviors that a person may be carrying a weapon.
- Fear of being perceived as "crying wolf" can prevent the detection and reaction to danger.
- Pattern matching can make you much safer from dangerous individuals while improving your connection with those around and forcing you to become more aware of the needs of others.
- Pay attention and observe the subtle differences in human behaviors that can indicate danger, and be prepared to act.
- Be aware that criminals often use these same methods to detect vulnerable victims.
- Demonstrating a sense of personal awareness can mitigate the vulnerability of your position.
- "People detectors" can help prevent violence from happening to themselves and others.

For more about how you can use pattern matching and recognition, visit *www.SafeHavensInternational.org*.

BIBLIOGRAPHY

Beer, M., R. M. Jayson, V. E. Carter, and F. H. Kresse (1961). *Survey of escape training in the Air Force.* Wright-Patterson Air Force Base, OH: Air Research and Development Command.

de Becker, G. (1997). *The gift of fear and other survival signals that protect us from violence.* New York: Dell Publishing.

Dorn, M. (2012). Safe Topics: The first 30 seconds. Macon, GA: Safe Havens International.

Gladwell, M. (2005) *Blink: The Power of Thinking Without Thinking.* Boston: Beck Bay Books.

Klein, G. (1998). *Sources of power: How people make decisions.* Cambridge, MA: The MIT Press.

Roberto, M. A. (2009). *Know what you don't know: How great leaders prevent problems before they happen.* Upper Saddle River, NJ: Pearson Prentice Hall.

U.S. Department of Homeland Security. (2013). *Bomb making materials awareness program.* Retrieved from the website of the Department of Homeland security. Retrieved from *http://www.dhs.gov*

Winter, J. (2012). *Massacre suspect James Holmes' gun-range application drew red flag.* Retrieved from *http://www.foxnews.com*

CHAPTER THREE

SECURITY TECHNOLOGIES AND HOW THEY AFFECT YOU

How to understand the amazing power as well as the limitations of security technologies.

On March 12, 2005, a man awaiting a retrial on rape charges was brought from his cell to a changing room outside a courtroom in Atlanta, Georgia. He suddenly attacked a deputy, seriously wounding her and taking her gun. He then went on a spree, killing a judge and a court reporter in the courtroom and a sheriff's deputy on the steps of the courthouse. In a furious manhunt that was featured on *America's Most Wanted,* he stole five cars, killed a federal agent, and held a woman hostage in her own home. He was eventually taken back into custody (Roh, 2005). He was convicted of four counts of first-degree murder and various other charges and is currently serving consecutive life sentences without the possibility of parole.

On April 15, 2013, the Boston Marathon was in full swing, with hundreds of people crossing the finish line and thousands more close behind. An explosion quickly shattered the exuberant mood—a mood so euphoric that some did not immediately recognize the sound as a bomb. The blast rocked the area, knocked down runners, and caused mass confusion. Seconds later, another explosion occurred a few hundred feet away. First responders and nearby citizens had reflexively rushed into the chaos to provide first aid and comfort to those who had been wounded. When the air cleared and the aftermath was assessed, the two explosions had killed three people and wounded 264 others (Kotz, 2013). The nation recoiled in horror as the events unfolded live on the news and social media. The world was given a play-by-play account through nonstop Twitter posts. The FBI and local law enforcement agencies worked together to identify the suspected attackers by releasing surveillance camera footage through media outlets—this was one of the first well-publicized uses of crowdsourcing to increase the speed of response to a mass casualty assault. In the subsequent manhunt and shootouts, one of the suspects was killed and the other taken into custody (Morales, 2013).

In both cases, technology played a key role in bringing the perpetrators to justice. But security technologies also failed to prevent either incident. We have seen this type of dynamic in many tragedies such as the London subway bombing. This is a key distinction and a primary reason for our writing this chapter. When considering how much you can rely on security technology to protect you, you need to have realistic expectations. Modern security technologies are nothing short of amazing and can, without question, make you safer. But these technologies are highly dependent on human operators and—like all protective measures—there are limitations.

The history of humanity is one of developing technologies to enhance and extend our senses as a means of survival. Early man would scatter rocks and dried leaves at the mouth of a cave to warn him of intruders, and nomadic tribes all over the world learned to observe the behavior of animals as early warning systems for predatory threats. Each day there are announcements of new developments in ever more sophisticated and intelligent security technology. As we rely more and more on computers to help keep us safe, it is important that we, as the human operators of this security technology and the people being protected by it, understand that tools are sometimes only as good as the skills of the person in control. Furthermore, the success of the operator often depends on the support and cooperation of those being protected. Studies of gas station robberies in Florida in the 1990s showed that the most important factor in the reduction of injury during armed robbery was the level of training of staff members rather than the specific types of equipment or technology in use (Atlas, 2013).

The events of September 11, 2001, are a stark reminder that even sophisticated security programs have gaps that must be continuously identified and addressed. It is not always possible to detect and correct all vulnerabilities. This means that it is even more important to understand where security technologies must be supported by human vigilance. Knowing how you can benefit from security technology and ways to increase the benefits of security investments can dramatically enhance your personal level of safety.

This chapter will also show how technologies should complement, rather than replace, our human senses when it comes to judgment and decision making. By understanding the benefits and limitations of cameras, metal detectors, and other security technologies, you can develop a more accurate view while avoiding a false sense of security. By learning to identify common gaps in security that can affect your safety, you will also be better able to make decisions based on an understanding of the level of safety at an event or location. This information can also help decision makers for organizations provide the types of leadership required to make security technologies more effective.

Technology Has Its Limits

A woman in New Jersey wanted to keep an eye on her babysitter, so she decided to install a "nanny cam" in her living room. During the day, a man broke into her apartment and began stealing things from her house before attacking her. In the end, the camera did not protect her from a vicious assault, but it did create a valuable record of the assault that was used to apprehend the thief (Rosenbaum, 2013). As this case shows, most security technology is passive. That means it operates without acting on its environment unless a human operator is actively controlling the technology. This is important as the actual purpose of many security technologies is to enhance our senses, not replace them.

At our nonprofit school safety center, we are sometimes asked by schools to perform a red team assessment—also known as a penetration test. In this type of assessment, our analysts try to breach the security of a school or other facility as a way of evaluating the effectiveness of the school's security measures. Most commonly, our analysts are able to simulate the theft of laptop computers, LCD projectors, master keys, employee identification cards, purses, car keys, vehicles (including school buses), and sensitive records with student and employee information. When asked to do so by our clients, we also conduct what are known as passive, nonthreatening simulated abductions of students. This means our analysts simulate an attempt to persuade students to go with us.

During this type of assessment at a client school district, one of our analysts was able to successfully "steal" more than 100 laptop computers, two maintenance trucks, two farm tractors, and 14 school children from 39 schools over an eight-day period of time, even though the district had invested in security cameras, proximity card readers for exterior doors, and buzzer access systems for entrances. Despite these tools, the practices of the people operating the technologies allowed our analysts to routinely beat these systems. These are relatively typical findings for schools where there has been a heavy investment in security technology but inadequate training of school employees. Although security technology can make it harder for an aggressor, nothing beats a combination of good physical security and an effective culture of security among the people who are being protected.

Erin and Abe's attack might have gone slightly differently if they had been able to effectively use one security technology they had at their disposal. When Erin, Judy, and the other two women ran for safety, they left their cell phones in the living room. Retreating to safe spaces without their phones meant that no one was able to call 911 until after the attack was over. Though not every technology is right for each situation, you should think about what tools and technologies you might have available and how they could help you during an emergency. Being ready to use them and knowing where they are located as a daily habit can be critical when seconds count.

In contrast, closed-circuit television (CCTV) cameras would likely not have provided a deterrent in Erin and Abe's attack. Security cameras have limitations for larger organizations as well. In our expert witness work, we routinely see instances where security camera footage is used in litigation *against* the organization that installed the cameras in the first place. For example, in school safety lawsuits, it is very common for security camera footage to be used to prove that students were not being properly supervised when an incident occurred. Schools that install millions of dollars in security camera equipment but do not provide formal training on techniques of effective student supervision are not only more likely to experience safety incidents but to be successfully litigated as well. It is also common to find metal detectors that have been purchased and installed but not used, as in the case of at least one school where a shooting occurred (Sprink, 2013). We are not averse to security technologies; however, we feel that it can be a mistake to invest money in them without also implementing the free strategies that have been proven to reduce crime or prevent it altogether.

Things to Consider When Using Security Technology

Intrusion alarms are becoming increasingly popular as technology costs decrease and more people seek to defend their properties against burglaries as well as armed robberies and other violent crimes. Intrusion alarms use various detection mechanisms like audio-, motion-, or magnetic-based sensors to detect unauthorized people entering an area. The simplest systems create an audible alarm that alerts anyone within a certain distance that an unauthorized entry has been made. Like a car alarm, these systems are designed to persuade the trespasser to leave while at the same time notifying bystanders of the breach. More advanced systems are monitored by dispatchers who alert security, police, or fire personnel to respond appropriately. This monitoring typically requires a setup cost and a recurring monthly fee.

When evaluating alarm systems, a key feature to consider is the specific notification process used. For example, if you have a duress button in your work area, where does it send the alarm signal to when you press it? In some facilities, internal security personnel or on-site police officers are automatically dispatched to the location of the duress button. In other instances, an alarm company must call 911 and request that local law enforcement officers be dispatched. It is also relatively common for duress buttons to be set up where they are monitored by on-site supervisory staff during normal business hours with no monitoring once these personnel are gone for the day. This can easily result in a situation where a person believes he or she has summoned assistance, whereas in reality no help is on the way.

Training for employees on *when* to use duress buttons is also critical. In our security assessments, we routinely find that employees have never been given any instructions on when and how to use duress buttons. For example, many employees are never told that they should also call for help by radio and/or telephone as soon as possible, since most duress buttons do not convey any information other than that a person is in distress at a specific location. There are however, some very robust technologies that combine audio and even video monitoring with duress buttons. For example, some systems activate cameras when a duress button is pressed. This allows a dispatcher in a remote location to observe the situation via live audio/video feed. Some of these technologies even allow police officers to listen to the audio feed while they are en route.

Modern education technology is also making it easier to provide this capability for schools. Several of the voice amplification systems that are becoming ever more common in classrooms provide teachers with a pendant to amplify their voice so students in the back of the room can hear them better. Giving a portable and practical personal amplification system to teachers has been shown to improve test scores and to provide an audio feed that can allow the school's front office or security personnel to hear what is said in the room in an emergency via the pendant microphone. Some systems can also integrate classroom or office duress button capability with live camera feeds with this same functionality.

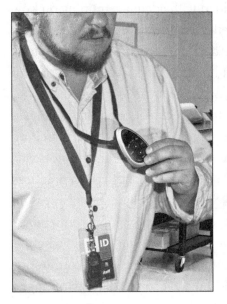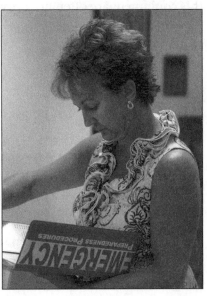

Pendant: There are a variety of tools available to make us safer, like this communication pendant that features an emergency duress button that instantly calls for help, letting emergency responders hear a live audio feed. These tools are also proven to improve test scores in schools when used to amplify a teacher's voice when coupled with a smartboard. Training on how to use this equipment—and on basic emergency procedures—is crucial to success in any crisis.
Photos: Rachel Wilson

Using an alarm company also requires at least some basic training for those who will operate the equipment. There are access codes, duress codes, and processes for arming and disarming the system. Many alarm systems also have a duress button feature—commonly called a panic button. As with any complex piece of equipment, the more control and options there are, the more chances there are for problems to arise because of user error. Users may input incorrect codes, forget code words, accidentally press the duress button without realizing it, or forget to arm the system altogether. It is important that all users practice frequently to lessen the probability of user error.

Many organizations now use camera and audio monitoring systems combined with a door buzzer to help screen visitors. As with other types of security technologies, the people who are expected to operate this equipment are often not provided with adequate training on how these systems can be used most effectively. This results in staff having to make many uncomfortable decisions when screening visitors. People who use such systems should be provided with some form of guidance through policy, training, and/or instructional video.

Pattern matching can be used to help detect potentially dangerous people during the visitor screening process. As pattern matching empowers people to look for patterns of behavior that are not congruent to a situation, effective staff and visitor identification practices can make it much easier for employees to spot a dangerous person. In addition, there are some very specific indicators of potential danger that you can look and listen for when screening visitors, whether it is at work, while you are on vacation, or at home. Most commonly, people who screen visitors should be alert to indications of anger, intoxication, and mental instability.

Advanced security systems allow users to gain access to and control the system via a smartphone or a tablet, allowing the user greater flexibility. However, this also increases the likelihood of someone "hacking" into your system using these devices, giving them access to your home or place of work. Currently, cell phones are often among the easiest devices to hack. In July 2013, a group of "white-hat" hackers demonstrated that commercially available equipment with a cost of less than $300 could be used to gain complete access to any cell phone within 40 feet (Sydell, 2013). Even though there will always be vulnerabilities, you should take steps to make these types of breaches more difficult. Make sure to follow or exceed the password recommendations of the alarm system's manufacturer. Consider purchasing improved security features or services for your mobile device as they become available, particularly if you can access sensitive information and/or control security systems through your device. If you frequently access the Internet on public networks using your mobile device or a laptop, consider using a virtual private network (VPN) service to provide a layer of security between your computer and third parties.

On a more basic level, smoke, fire, and carbon monoxide detectors should be in every home. These devices detect dangerous elements in the atmosphere of your home and provide an audible tone to alert you to the presence of danger. These devices require proper placement and a power source. Most consumer-level detectors are battery operated and require regular replacement of the batteries, though some more advanced detectors like those integrated into alarm systems are powered directly from the building's power lines. An integrated smoke detector saved the life of a young man in Needham, Connecticut, when a refrigerator caught fire on the top floor of his parent's home while he was sleeping. He did not hear the alarms, but the system alerted the local fire department, and they responded in time to wake the young man up and put the fire out (Manning, 2012).

These devices are limited in that they rely on the homeowner to properly place them and continue to provide them with power or service if they are integrated into an alarm system. Too often, homeowners will forget to replace the batteries in a smoke detector, leaving themselves without warning if their home catches fire. Coauthor Steve Satterly learned that he had forgotten to change the batteries in his home's smoke detector one day in 2012. He was sitting in the living room reading, when his wife walked into the room and asked, "What's burning?" She walked into the kitchen and saw that a skillet was on fire because the burner had been left on. The fire was quickly put out, and afterwards the smoke detector was checked and the batteries replaced.

Satterly has since installed a new system that has the smoke detector tied into the home security system. This type of system often will provide an alert when the batteries are low, and again if the batteries die. This is especially important for Satterly, as he has a condition known as *anosmia*. People with anosmia have no sense of smell. For people with anosmia, smoke detectors and alarm systems are even more important as they cannot detect a fire as rapidly as most people. This is an excellent example of how various safety, security, and emergency preparedness technologies can help better protect people who have special needs or living situations. There are a number of excellent technologies that can help people who have increased vulnerabilities for any reason.

Weapons Screening Checkpoints

Many government facilities, sporting venues, businesses, and schools use metal detectors to screen people for guns, knives, and other contraband. Modern metal detectors are extremely effective at detecting the presence of metal on your person. However, the detection of metal does not always correlate to the presence of a weapon. As most readers have probably experienced, a significant percentage of people passing through metal detector checkpoints have to undergo additional screening because they have harmless metal on their person that sets off the detector. At the same time, the absence of an alarm from the metal detector does not mean that a person is not armed. Operator error, sensitivity settings, plastic yet lethal weapons, and concealment methods all create limitations in the application of weapons screening technology in any setting.

Coauthors Michael Dorn and Chris Dorn have worked extensively with one of the world's largest metal detector manufacturers. Having an advanced knowledge of the proper and improper applications of this type of equipment, along with the technical limitations of this technology and X-ray screening equipment, they frequently notice gaps in screening programs in foreign airports, event venues, and other locations where metal detectors are in use. During our red team assessments, we are frequently able to defeat security and successfully smuggle in weapons including firearms and knives through security screening checkpoints.

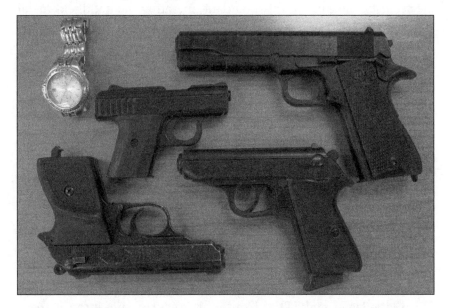

Guns: At a client's request, coauthor Michael Dorn was able to smuggle all of these replica firearms through an improperly operated metal detector checkpoint during a security audit of the client's high-rise office building.
Photo: Michael Dorn

As with security cameras, we feel that metal detectors can be highly effective when used properly and appropriately supported by other security measures.

Effective entry point metal detection requires extensive support-ive measures. Entry point metal detection is most commonly used at airports, courthouses, and other facilities where people must be screened before being admitted. It is very common to see ineffective entry point metal detection that can easily be defeated. For example, if hand-carry items like purses or book bags are not checked by secu-rity X-ray screening, it is generally very easy to get a gun or other contraband through the checkpoint. This is because it is difficult to properly search these types of items by hand in a reasonable amount of time without security X-ray equipment.

Coauthor Chris Dorn experienced an example of entry point screening operator error while flying from Saigon to Quy Nhơn, Vietnam. At the security checkpoint, the attendant operating the handheld metal detector was wearing a heavy military uniform with large brass buttons on the front of the jacket. The handheld metal detector repeatedly set off an alarm tone because of the brass buttons on the operator's jacket. Perhaps because of this interference, or possibly because of a misunderstanding of how to use the equipment, the operator completely ignored the signal from the metal detector and did not perform any additional screening before clearing Dorn to pass.

In other instances, offenders have beaten metal detector checkpoints by simply bypassing them. For example, we have conducted assessments at several schools where elaborate weapons screening checkpoints are stationed at the front doors but several other exterior doors of the school are left unlocked every school day so students can get to and from portable classrooms outside the school. This blatant gap makes the front entry security measures at these schools unreliable. Not surprisingly, the principal at one of these schools reported that a student had recently been caught with a handgun in the school.

Another common vulnerability for metal detection checkpoints is the security of the checkpoint itself. Any checkpoint that is not in some way protected by armed security or law enforcement personnel can be easily defeated by anyone with a gun who is willing to use it. This was demonstrated in the Red Lake Reservation High School shooting where the aggressor shot and killed an unarmed security officer to defeat a metal detection checkpoint before killing a number of staff and students (Alert system fell, 2005).

Properly operated weapons screening checkpoints can be extremely effective when they are properly staffed and are supported by appropriate physical security measures. You should always consider the possibility that a checkpoint can be beaten and avoid lulling yourself into a false sense of security because you were screened as you entered a concert, museum, or office building. Our analysts have noted that employees who work in facilities with entry point weapons screening often have an assumption of safety that could contribute to a tragedy. For example, while conducting a school security assessment for one of the nation's largest school districts, we ran controlled simulations of crisis simulations using dynamic videos with employees from each school. We found that employees we tested were typically unable to respond to any scenario we posed that included a person with a gun, knife, hammer, crowbar, or other weapon.

Employees repeatedly told us that the scenarios depicted were impossible because students and visitors had to pass through a metal detection checkpoint to enter the building. Our analysts knew that we had already proven that anyone could easily get a weapon into each of the schools we assessed due to a variety of security gaps. Most typically, that we found exterior doors propped open at almost every one of the schools during our assessments. We also noted that numerous students had been caught with weapons after they had passed through these same checkpoints, and there have been shootings in schools with this type of entry point screening. As we explore the effects of stress on the human mind and body, it will become apparent how the inability of these employees to respond to video simulations would be significantly higher under the stress of an actual crisis. Finally, as the incident in the Georgia Courthouse illustrates, a mass casualty shooting can still occur in a high-security environment even where effective weapons screening is in place (McDonald, 2008).

Integrating Technology into Your Safety Plans

In Chapter One, you read about how to conduct an assessment of your personal surroundings. When you do an assessment at your home, workplace, or other setting, you will identify risks that should be considered and addressed. Your technology strategy can then be developed with the goal of addressing those risks and either preventing them or helping you to respond more effectively when those risks materialize. The use of technology, in this regard, is a "force multiplier." This is a term used in the military to describe something that strengthens your capabilities. A force multiplier is not a force replacement. Your plan should include the use of technology to multiply your capabilities of protecting yourself, but it will also be important to include contingencies for the potential loss of technology. During major disasters like hurricane Katrina and super storm Sandy, utility networks, government services, and cell phone services experienced severe outages and delays in service for days and, in some cases, weeks.

This is why is it important to make the assessment process a natural part of what you do, even in rapidly evolving situations. This is where you can identify how security technology can help and when it might have vulnerabilities. After that, it becomes a matter of problem solving. An important point here is that if you learn to assess your surroundings naturally as part of what you do every day, assessing and reacting will become a natural behavior, much like driving a car or riding a bicycle. When done properly, this should reduce, rather than increase, your fear. We will discuss many terrible events in this book as teaching tools, but remember that survival is just as integral to human nature as violence. Man has been committing rape, murder, and child abuse since before written records were created. Some men and women will always victimize others if they are allowed to do so. But it is often possible to counter this reality. Keeping this perspective while we take reasonable steps to protect ourselves can afford you a sense of safety and control to replace the fear that can change who we are if we are not careful.

Conclusion

Technology has its place in the big picture of security and protection from those who wish to harm you. However, safety technology is not infallible. It is up to you to understand technology so it can become a force multiplier. That understanding will also prevent you from becoming too reliant on the technology itself, since technology is usually passive. It will not actively respond to an aggressor without human assistance. It can detect when unauthorized entry has occurred, and it can sometimes even summon assistance, but the presence of the technology itself provides no guarantee that a determined attacker will be prevented from committing acts of crime or violence.

Keep your expectations about technology realistic, and remember to rely primarily on your most powerful protective tool, your brain. There is no security technology that works as fast as the properly prepared human brain to detect and react to the many types of dangerous situations that we can encounter. A healthy combination of excellent security technology and alert and properly prepared people can be an excellent defense against tragedy.

Key Points in Chapter Three

- Technologies are highly dependent on human operators and are only as good as the skills, equipment, and authority of the person who is in control.
- Learn to seek out, identify, and address common gaps in security that can affect your safety.
- While security technology can make it harder for a person to commit a criminal act, nothing beats a combination of good physical security and an effective culture of security among the people who are being protected.
- Think about what tools and technologies you might have available to you and how they could help you during an emergency.
- Modern metal detectors are extremely effective at detecting the presence of metal on your person; however, the detection of metal does not always correlate to the presence of a weapon.
- Consider the possibility that a checkpoint can be beaten, and avoid lulling yourself into a false sense of security. The presence of the technology itself provides no guarantee that a determined attacker will be prevented from committing acts of crime or violence.
- Include contingencies for the potential loss of technology.

BIBLIOGRAPHY

Alert system fell silent during Red Lake school shooting. (2005). PostBulletin.
com. Retrieved from *http://www.postbulletin.com/alert-system-fell-
silent-during-red-lake-school-shooting/article_8d3095d4-38a7-58b8-84f0-
4e659f963f56.html?mode=jqm*

Atlas, R. I. (2013). *21st century security and CPTED: Designing for critical
infrastructure protection and crime prevention (2nd ed.).* Boca Raton, FL:
CRC Press.

Kotz, D. (2013). Injury toll from Marathon bombs reduced to 264. *The Boston
Globe.* Retrieved from *http://www.bostonglobe.com/lifestyle/healthwellness/
2013/04/23/number-injured-marathon-bombing revised downward/
NRpaz5mmvGquP7KMA6XsIK/story.html*

Manning, B. (2012). Alarm system may have saved man's life in Pine Street
fire. *Needham Patch.* Retrieved from *http://needham.patch.com/groups/
police-and-fire/p/alarm-system-may-have-saved-man-s-life-in-pine-street-fire*

McDonald, G. L., and R. R. McDonald. (2008). Courthouse shooting case opens
with audiotape of gunshots. *Law.com.* Retrieved from *http://www.law.com/jsp/
article.jsp?id=1202424720420*

Morales, D. B., and L. M. Moralesa. (2013). Boston Marathon bombing suspects
caught on camera, FBI seeks help in identifying them. *Daily News.* Retrieved
from *http://www.nydailynews.com/news/national/tiny-victim-bombing-
recovering-article-1.1320266*

Roh, J. (2005). Judge, two others killed in courthouse shooting. *FoxNews.com.*
Retrieved from *http://www.foxnews.com/story/2005/03/12/judge-two-others-
killed-in-courthouse-shooting/*

Rosenbaum, S. (2013). Suspect in nanny-cam beating pleads not guilty. U.S.
News on NBCNews.com. Retrieved from *http://usnews.nbcnews.com/
_news/2013/07/02/19251258-suspect-in-nanny-cam-beating-pleads-not-guilty*

Sprink, M. K. G., and J. Sprink. (2013). APS: Metal detectors "not operable" on
day of school shooting. *Atlanta Journal Constitution.* Retrieved from *http://
www.ajc.com/news/news/crime-law/police-atlanta-school-shooting-gang-re-
lated/nWC9W/*

Sydell, L. (2013). How hackers tapped into my cellphone for less than $300.
All Tech Considered. Retrieved from *http://www.npr.org/blogs/
alltechconsidered/2013/07/15/201490397/How-Hackers-Tapped-Into-My-
Verizon-Cellphone-For-250*

CHAPTER FOUR

MITIGATION—REDUCING THE NEGATIVE IMPACT OF CRISIS SITUATIONS

Mitigation—reducing the negative impact of events that either cannot be prevented or occur in spite of prevention efforts.

Tornados, armed robberies, school violence, and flooding: what do these risks have in common? They are each almost impossible to prevent with 100 percent certainty. What can we do when faced with threats like these that can bring death and destruction with little warning?

At Riley Children's Hospital, a nationally recognized children's hospital in Indianapolis, Indiana, employees are given breaks on their insurance premiums if they meet certain benchmarks like overall weight, body-fat index, and abstinence from tobacco. This provides employees the economic incentive to develop healthier lifestyles, leading to reduced use of the insurance plan that the hospital offers its employees.

In a small town in Oklahoma, a new home is being built. "Tornado straps" are applied where the ceiling joists meet the wall joists. This will help prevent high winds from lifting the roof off of the walls, which could cause the walls to collapse. Connecting the walls to the foundation, using wind-resistant shingles and thicker vinyl siding can all reduce the damage to severe winds (Gardella, 2011). A shelter is also being constructed in the ground a short distance away from the house, which could make the difference between life and death in a tornado.

An office manager seeks the advice of his sheriff's department crime prevention unit. A sheriff's deputy visits his business and suggests that a safe room be created from an existing storage room. The deputy points out that the room is of cement block construction, has a solid wood door and a sturdy lock, and is located close to the main office. The deputy suggests that the room be cleaned up to create more space, that a phone line be added, and that employees be taught how to quickly retreat to the room, lock the door, and call 911 in an emergency.

In a school, a bullying prevention program is implemented, teaching students what bullying looks like and giving them a procedure to anonymously report it. This program is helpful to students who experience bullying, which cannot be prevented completely. When bullying occurs, the impact of the bully is reduced by rapid, effective intervention, with consequences for the bully and support for the victim.

A Midwestern town is flooded every spring when melting snow and spring rains cause the nearby river to overflow its banks. The town receives state and federal funding to build a series of levees along the river. These levees help contain the rising floodwaters and direct them away from the town, saving the town hundreds of thousands of dollars a year in floodwater rescue and recovery activities.

What is the common thread in all of these stories? They each depict the concept of mitigation: "the effort to reduce loss of life and property by lessening the impact of disasters" (What is, 2013). Any event or emergency that causes disruption to you—whether it be socially or medically or to your property—is considered a "hazard" in emergency management terms. Mitigation focuses on those measures that will lessen or remove the impact of a hazard after it occurs. Mitigation in this sense is a concept developed by the field of emergency management. Mitigation focuses on actions you take now to lessen future impacts. Prevention is the ideal; however, mitigation is very important for those situations we cannot prevent, like a tornado. Mitigation is also important for those situations that take place in spite of our best prevention efforts, like the shooting in the workplace. Because of the focus on preincident actions, mitigation measures are often part of or blended with actions we take to prevent or prepare for hazards.

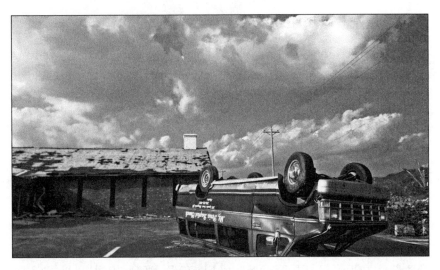

Tornado damage: Each year we are reminded of the critical importance of being prepared for natural disasters. This is the aftermath of the 175mph winds of an F4 tornado that killed 8 people and injured more than 30 others in Ringgold, Georgia on April 27, 2011.
Photo: Chris Dorn

Because mitigation helps us once an incident takes place, it is not as "clean" as prevention, where there may be clear-cut examples of incidents that are averted. Mitigation efforts might reduce, but not eliminate, the number of fatalities in a shooting. A rapidly implemented lockdown can reduce the opportunity for an aggressor to shoot victims. As with any strategy, you have to be prepared to lockdown fast enough. A delay in locking down is like closing the door on a submarine when you are fifty feet underwater. Many strategies require mental and physical preparedness to act.

This chapter will help you understand the role of mitigation at home, work, or wherever you may face risk. It will also demonstrate the money-saving aspects of mitigation. Two main forms of mitigation, technical and social, will be explained and demonstrated. While we will share numerous examples of mitigation, it is important to remember that your use of mitigation will be dependent on specific hazards and the specific physical aspects of the environment. There is no such thing as a one-size-fits-all mitigation strategy.

Technical Approaches

Mitigation requires a variety of technical approaches. Many of these involve design features that are physically built or created in a building or a space to mitigate an identified hazard. The examples of the home being built in Oklahoma and the levee being built in a Midwestern town illustrate this type of approach. The tornado straps help lessen the damage to a home by severe winds, and the shelter helps lessen the danger to the home's occupants. The levee reduces the potential flood damage to people or property in the town.

While mitigation is extremely important for a home, it can be particularly important for other settings including retail stores, businesses, schools, event venues, and places of worship. This is because these settings often have a much greater potential for mass casualty incidents because of the relatively large populations that use them, multiplying the number of lives that could be affected. For example, many of our more advanced school clients have built-in shutoff switches that allow one-step shutdown of air-handling units. This allows a school principal to reduce the flow of air into the school if there is a hazardous materials incident nearby by pushing a button. This mitigation measure could be effective whether the incident was the result of a terrorist attack using chemicals or radiological components, or for the much more likely scenario of a train or truck accident.

In Chapter Three we discussed security technologies, which often serve as mitigation measures. For example, a home alarm system helps to mitigate against death or injuries from fire or smoke inhalation. A simple weather radio can mitigate against injury or death by providing you with enough warning to get to a shelter or a safe area in your home if there is a tornado.

The technical approach to mitigation is straightforward: build or create things that eliminate or reduce the negative impact of a crisis.

Identify hazards and then come up with ways to eliminate or reduce the potential impact on you and your community. There can be costs involved, but remember, any money you invest now will save you money later if the hazard manifests itself. There is even a return on investment in mitigation measures. According to a study by the Hazard Mitigation Council, every $1 spent in mitigation measures saves $4 in crisis response costs (Eguchi et al., 2005)

Social Approach

The social approach to mitigation is more complex because it involves people. The social approach to mitigation works by strengthening social structures, which increases resiliency for the group as a whole during an emergency. This, in turn, reduces the overall impact of those emergencies (Kapucu, 2012, p. 40). The goal of the social approach is to increase awareness of hazards and their nature and share ways to reduce the potential impact of each hazard. The social approach also focuses on increasing the adaptability and resiliency of those affected by a hazard. Leadership is usually necessary to convince others of the existence of the threat in the face of denial or ignorance of the real level of risk.

Let us start with a simple example in a family home. A mother has heard rumors about a rash of burglaries in the neighborhood. She meets with the family and shares what she has learned. They discuss ways to reduce the impact of a burglar getting into their house and ways to secure valuables in the house, making a mental note to not leave video cameras or laptop computers out where they can be seen through windows. These steps can either deter a burglar or cause them to take longer to enter the home or locate valuables.

The important step in this process was the communication between family members. This conversation can help lessen the impact of a hazard just by mentally simulating the event by thinking about it. This can be critical for any threat to a family, workforce, or social institution. With communication and leadership comes collaboration, which increases resilience.

The next step in the social process involves fostering improved understanding. Having become aware of the burglaries, the family in our example looked into the nature of the problem. They attended a neighborhood watch meeting where a local police officer shared some information developed from previous break-ins. From the meeting, people in the neighborhood got to know each other and became aware of threats in the community and ways to prevent and mitigate them. In addition, the neighborhood also started to develop a familiarity with the same police officers that will respond in the event of a crisis. This increased the overall understanding of each role in the community, which improves resiliency and can reduce the group impact of any hazard.

The social approach then informs the technical approach. Having one without the other is not as effective as combining the two. In this case, installing simple pins in each window might make it more difficult to break into the house. While this approach will not stop a determined burglar, it will slow the burglar down, reducing the number of items he can steal. This approach also increases the chances the burglar will be caught and valuables recovered.

This hypothetical family is a simple, idealized example, but it demonstrates the need to involve all stakeholders in mitigation. In your home, you want to involve your family. At work, you want to involve your coworkers. Anyone who would be affected by the hazard should be involved in mitigating against it.

Often, the greatest obstacle to the social approach is denial. This is because there is a distinct human tendency to engage in denial. Sometimes teachers do not accept that bullying occurs in their schools, and never "buy in" to bullying mitigation efforts. A strong system to educate staff on the realities and the consequences of bullying is necessary to help overcome this sort of denial. Looking back to our hypothetical family, people often fail to realize the real threat level in their own neighborhood when it comes to burglaries or violent crime. As a result, they do not actively participate in community meetings like the one we described.

Erin and Abe had been friends with their attacker and his wife before the attack. His behavior that day did not fit with his prior behavior, and they could not reconcile the complete difference between the two people they had encountered. This is a classic example of denial. Rather than accept the reality of what happened, they chose to provide the simplistic explanation that the attacker "just snapped." We are all prone to this common reaction to events that our brain cannot reconcile with patterns that it recognizes.

Denial can be a very powerful barrier to survival. Psychologically speaking, it is easier to be in denial than it is to see the signs of impending violence so that we can take action. This can lead to problems, as Grossman explains in the context of a police officer who does not carry a gun while off duty:

> Denial kills you twice; It kills you once, at your moment of truth, when you are not physically prepared: You didn't bring your gun; you didn't train. Your only defense was wishful thinking. Hope is not a strategy. Denial kills you a second time because even if you do physically survive, you are psychologically shattered by fear, helplessness, horror and shame at your moment of truth. (Grossman and Christensen, 2011)

Denial is an obstacle to all facets of emergency management at any level. We must set aside denial so that we will not die twice.

Conclusion

Like a police officer who carries a backup gun in case the primary weapon is taken from him or her or malfunctions, mitigation measures can provide a backup mechanism to save your life. When properly applied and the trap of denial is avoided, we can significantly reduce the potential for loss of life during a life or death situation.

Key Points in Chapter Four

- It is important to focus on prevention, but we should also include mitigation as a critical life-saving approach.

- Mitigation is distinct from prevention and includes both social and technical measures taken to eliminate a threat or reduce its impact.
- The use of mitigation will be dependent on a specific hazard and the physical aspects of the environment. Identify hazards and then come up with a plan to diminish the threat or reduce its potential impact.
- Through communication and leadership comes collaboration, which increases resilience.
- Denial can cloud our ability to prevent or mitigate against risk. It is easier to be in denial than it is to see the signs of impending violence, and it is often easier to be in denial of warning signs in people we know and like.
- Be aware of your surroundings and the real threats you are vulnerable to.
- Share information with your family, neighbors, and coworkers, work on a plan, and be ready to take action.

BIBLIOGRAPHY

Eguchi, R., C. Taylor, A. Rose, K. Porter, and T. McLane. (2005). *Natural hazard mitigation saves: An independent study to assess future savings from mitigation activities.* Washington, DC: National Institute of Building Sciences. Retrieved from *http://c.ymcdn.com/sites/www.nibs.org/ resource/resmgr/MMC/hms_vol1.pdf*

Gardella, L. M., and R. Gardella. (2011). Tornado-proofing homes? $1 straps would help. *Weather on NBCNews.* Retrieved from *http://www.nbcnews.com/ id/43991294/ns/weather/t/tornado-proofing-homes-straps-would-help/ #.UdSuXFOvt7Y*

Grossman, D., and L. W. Christensen. (2011, July 10). On combat: The psychology and physiology of deadly conflict in war and peace (Kindle Locations 3927-3930). Human Factor Research Group, Inc. Kindle Edition.

Guide for developing high-quality emergency operations plans for institutions of higher education. (2013). Washington, DC: U.S. Department of Education.

Kapucu, N. (2012). *Managing emergencies and crises.* Burlington, VT: Jones and Bartlett Learning.

What is mitigation? (2013). Retrieved June 18, 2013, from *http://www.fema.gov/ what-mitigation*

CHAPTER FIVE

KNOWING THE SIGNS OF VIOLENCE

Or how you can detect potentially dangerous people.

The woman tested the condo door and found it unlocked. She quietly opened it and walked through the dark kitchen to the bedroom door. She opened it to see her victim asleep in bed. The woman gazed at her, thinking of past arguments. She thought, "She's just like the others, always out to get me. She'll pay." She pulled out a handgun and pointed it at her target. She poked her prey in the nose, and just as the woman woke up, she pulled the trigger. She turned and left the condo, heading for her former workplace, a postal processing center in Goleta, California.

She went on to kill five more people before shooting herself. This incident occurred on January 30, 2006, and is believed to have been the deadliest act of workplace violence by a woman to date (Kasindorf, 2006). When an event like this happens, people often say that the killer "just snapped." In the story of Abe and Erin, denial caused them to miss several warning signs. It is often easier to be in denial of warning signs in people we know and like.

Mary Tyler, an expert on workplace violence, tells us, "The cases we know about, it's not usually a sudden snap. Usually, the person is badly depressed and feels hopeless. They probably feel angry, frustrated. They've probably been going downhill in their life for a while," she said. "They may have been talking about weapons and violent subjects" (Kasindorf, 2006). Before people become violent, they often provide others with signs that they are on a path—or continuum—of violence. In this chapter, we will explore this continuum and how we can use this as a practical way to prevent violence.

The Continuum of Violence

Dr. Stephen Holmes and Dr. Richard Holmes are renowned for their work in forensic psychology and behavioral analysis. Their textbooks are a standard reference for forensic psychology, and their research has helped police understand the minds of serial killers, mass murderers, and sexual predators. They identified the continuum of violence as a path of escalation from low to high.

This continuum has three levels: Intimidation, Escalation, and Further Escalation (Holmes and Holmes, 2001). The continuum of violence is not smooth or regular. It is not as simple as a person showing a series of signs in a specific order. A person might seem to jump from intimidation to further escalation rapidly, or someone might show signs of escalation without posing a danger to others or ever showing signs in the other two areas. You should look for a change in normal behavior, with clusters of concerning behaviors. This is even more likely after a "trigger," or an emotional event.

In Gavin de Becker's best-selling book *The Gift of Fear* (1997), he mentions the work of Park Dietz, a renowned forensic psychologist and an expert on violence. Dietz wrote that stories about violence are "littered with reports, letters, memoranda, and recollections that show people felt uncomfortable, threatened, intimidated, violated and unsafe because of the very person who later committed atrocious acts of violence" (de Becker, 1997, p. 177). One of the themes of Becker's book is trusting your instincts. If someone's behavior bothers you, consider why it bothers you, and bring it to the attention of someone who can do something about it.

Looking into someone's behavior is useless unless you know what that behavior means. The continuum of violence can provide context for a person's behavior, but it is not predictive. A person who exhibits these signs will not necessarily become violent, but they are red flags that can indicate someone poses a threat.

LEVEL ONE—INTIMIDATION

This lowest level is the one most frequently seen. Remember that exhibiting these signs does not mean that a person will become a killer, but people who show these signs are certainly not pleasant to be around (Holmes and Holmes, 2001):

- Refusing to cooperate with authority
- Spreading rumors and gossip to harm others
- Constantly arguing with others
- Constant belligerence or swearing at others
- Making unwelcome sexual comments

Generally, it is best to bring these behaviors to the attention of someone who can help. If the subject were a coworker, your employer or your human resources department would be appropriate. If the person is a family member, you may need to seek professional help from a counselor or therapist.

LEVEL TWO—ESCALATION

People around this person will have feelings that range from dislike to unease. As the aggressor's behaviors escalate, it will become imperative that your supervisors, or others in authority, become aware of these behaviors (Holmes and Holmes, 2001):

- Increasing arguments with others
- Refusal to obey policies and procedures
- Sabotaging equipment or stealing property for revenge
- Verbalizing their wishes to harm others
- Sending unwanted sexual notes
- Having a "me versus them" mentality

These individuals will not be pleasant to be around, and most people will seek to avoid them. If they are not removed from the others or receive help, their behavior could quickly escalate further. We know from de Becker that if you are feeling threatened or intimidated, there are probably real reasons. Look for those reasons, investigate, and take action if appropriate.

LEVEL THREE—FURTHER ESCALATION

A person who exhibits these behaviors is dangerous. The person is already committing forms of violence, or such behaviors are imminent (Holmes and Holmes, 2001). The person may display frequent displays of anger resulting in (Holmes and Holmes, 2001):

- Recurrent suicidal threats
- Recurrent physical fights
- Destruction of property
- Use of weapons to harm others
- Commission of murder/rape/arson

If you become aware that someone is exhibiting these signs, you should notify the police. Chances are they may already be aware of some of these activities, but do not assume anything. In some cases, a person may exhibit separate signs in different locations, such as at work, social gatherings, church, or local businesses. De Becker teaches us that our minds often give us early warning signs of danger so it is important to coordinate and pool our resources when dealing with dangerous individuals.

Intoxication, Dangerous Mental Illness, and Anger

These three basic conditions affect people's behavior so much and occur with such frequency that they should be seen as possible warning signs when you observe them. In some cases, two or more of these conditions are present when an attack occurs. Not everyone who is angry is dangerous, but a lot of people end up in prison for things they did to other people when they were mad. Similarly, even though many people have abused alcohol or controlled substances without ever becoming violent, it is not hard to find inmates who became violent while they were under the influence of drugs and/or alcohol and did something to cause their incarceration. Most people who are mentally ill are not dangerous; however, dangerously mentally ill individuals have carried out some of our most horrific acts of violence such as the deadly bombing that left more than 40 children and educators dead at the Bath School in 1927.

Fortunately, there are proven training programs that can dramatically reduce the odds that you will be harmed by someone who is angry. Some of our clients have achieved dramatic reductions in injuries to employees through formal training in evidence-based de-escalation techniques. By training staff to use proven approaches to calming people who are upset, an organization can significantly reduce the chances that employees will be physically attacked by people who are angry. A number of other approaches we have discussed in this book can help increase the chances that you will spot danger and react with the speed necessary to prevent an attack. For example, recognizing the potential for danger when you encounter someone who is angry, intoxicated, or dangerously mentally ill.

Stranger Danger

In the opening chapter of *The Gift of Fear*, Gavin de Becker recounts the story of a woman who returned home from a shopping trip carrying several heavy shopping bags. After dropping one of her bags, she was approached by a man who insisted on helping her carry her bags to her apartment despite her repeated refusals for help. After reaching her apartment, he invited himself inside and raped her for three hours. After sensing that he was going to kill her before leaving, she managed to escape just in time to save her life. She later learned that the man had killed one of his other victims. Having ignored her intuition once before being raped, she managed to escape with her life because of choosing to follow her intuition when the rapist said "I promise, I'm not going to hurt you"—an example of what de Becker refers to as the "Unsolicited Promise" (de Becker, 1997).

In analyzing this story, de Becker identified a series of warning signs that are common signs of potentially dangerous manipulation. Sometimes manipulation is benign. Children manipulate parents, and we all seek to manipulate others to some degree to get what we want. However, there are predators who rely heavily on manipulation. Often, the signs of manipulation make us uncomfortable. We frequently discount these feelings, leaving us open to techniques intended to disarm our defenses. *The Gift of Fear* describes seven signs that a person is trying to manipulate you. Depending on the context, they can spell out danger.

Signs of Potentially Dangerous Manipulation (Chapter 4, *The Gift of Fear*)

- **"Forced Teaming"**: The manipulator invents a common purpose that doesn't exist by using words like "we" and "us" in relation to a real or invented goal. This makes it easier for the manipulator to invade personal space.
- **"Charm and Niceness"**: The manipulator charms us using niceness to erode our natural defense mechanisms.
- **"Too Many Details"**: Manipulators often add details beyond what is necessary to elude suspicion, and this can also cause us to tune out and let our guard down.
- **"Typecasting"**: Manipulators may challenge a victim to provoke a desired response; for example, a sexual predator may tell a child, "There is such a thing as being too independent," as a means to prompt rebellious behavior and lure a child closer.
- **"Loan-Sharking"**: Manipulators may do favors for us so we will feel pressured to give something in return or allow our personal space to be invaded.
- **"The Unsolicited Promise"**: A promise by a stranger without proper context is often a good signal that the person is up to no

good, for example: "If you let me use your phone I'll leave, *I prom-ise.*" Ask yourself, "What does this person offer if the promise is broken?"

- **Discounting the Word "No":** The manipulator who ignores repeated dismissal or refusals is exhibiting one of the most pow-erful warning signs of danger. A person who will not take "no" for an answer cares little for your wishes, which signals how little you mean to him. Such a person is definitely a manipulator.

In many cases, there are tangible signs of impending violence, but people often fail to recognize them or if they do, their brains are overcome by the power of denial and what is known as the brain's normalcy bias. When it comes to acts of violence, a proactive approach can make all the difference in recognizing danger rather than explaining it away until it is too late.

A person using these techniques will most likely be, at best, uncomfortable to be around and, at worst, a danger to your well-being. In the case of the woman described by de Becker in *The Gift of Fear,* her attacker exhibited each of these behaviors in the preparation and execution of his assault. Identify these signs in your everyday interaction with others. Knowing they are being used against you will cause them to lose power over you, and you will learn to trust your feelings about people, as you can explain why they are happening.

Most of us spend a lot of time around strangers. We interact with them at restaurants, theaters, amusement parks, and shopping malls. Even though most of the people we encounter in life mean us no harm, some do. In some cases, some people may be extremely dan-gerous. One of the best survival skills we can develop is the abil-ity to know when we are a potential target. We highly recommend de Becker's outstanding book *The Gift of Fear* for people who would like to learn more about how they can spot potentially dangerous people.

Beware the Child You Think You Know

It is difficult to apply the above warning signs to children. Their minds are not fully developed, and they see the world differently than adults. It is for this reason that police interviews with children are conducted differently than interviews with adults. The adults, at a different developmental level than children, will react differently to questions. The psychological and physiological cues we look for to help judge the meaning of what they are saying are different.

Children often give concrete, identifiable signs that they are in distress. Knowing those signs can help counter their words, which are often at odds with what they are doing. For example, a child may strike another child, and when asked, "What's wrong? Why did you do that?" the child will reply, "Nothing's wrong. I don't know why I did that." Often they are being truthful and may not understand why they did it. They lack the abstract thinking skills necessary to correctly use introspection. But there are behavioral signs that can provide you with early warnings of danger. They are divided into two categories—early warning signs that indicate we should be vigilant for more serious problems, and imminent warning signs that indicate an immediate risk to the child or others.

Early Warning Signs

Each of these signs depends heavily on the context and the person's normal behavior and personality, among other factors. These warning signs are some of the first indicators that a youth may be having issues and is progressing on the continuum of potentially harming himself/herself or others. The youth might warrant counseling or other types of acute intervention (Dorn and Dorn, 2008).

- Social withdrawal
- Excessive feelings of isolation, rejection, or being persecuted
- Being a victim of violence
- For students, low school interest and poor academics

- Expressions of violence in writing
- Uncontrolled anger
- Intolerance and prejudice
- Patterns of impulsive and chronic hitting
- Intimidation or bullying of others
- Chronic disciplinary issues
- History of violence, threats, or aggressive behavior
- Drug or alcohol abuse
- Affiliation with gangs or hate groups
- Access to firearms (in combination with other warning signs)

These signs should be seen as signals for you to seek help for the child. They are cries for help. Intervention at this stage may steer the child from violent behavior, but ignoring these signs may lead to imminent warning signs. Keep in mind that these are not necessarily indicators of violence but are more general signs of at-risk youth.

Imminent Warning Signs

Imminent warning signs are more urgent and require immediate intervention. If interventions in the early warning stages have not worked, if your child meets a new friend, or if a school has a transfer student, then these signs may appear without warning. You may still see early warning signs, since the earlier behaviors are likely to continue as the youth progresses into this stage.

Look for these behaviors to indicate at-risk youths who are at immediate risk of injuring themselves or others (Dorn and Dorn, 2008):

- Serious and violent fighting with peers and family
- Severe destruction of property
- Severe rage for seemingly minor reasons
- Detailed threats of lethal violence
- Possession/use of firearms and other weapons
- Self-injurious behaviors or threats/attempts at suicide

It is important to repeat that these are not necessarily warning signs of violence but warning signs of at-risk individuals. Many of these indicators have been incorporated into what are known as threat assessment programs that schools can use to identify potential threats before it is too late. Along with Deputy Chief Russell Bentley and school social worker Mitch Mitchell, coauthor Michael Dorn developed the concept of multidisciplinary threat assessment for schools in the early 1990s. The Bibb County Board of Education had extensive success with this program in preventing violence. Since then, these concepts have been developed and improved in the form of various more advanced models around the nation. Like the adult continuum of violence, these programs use particular warning signs along a continuum combined with multidisciplinary evaluation of the situation to determine the best course of action to help the student avoid dangerous behavior.

One of the most widely implemented is the Virginia Student Threat Assessment Guidelines, which has been rigorously evaluated over the course of 2 field trials and 4 controlled studies involving more than a thousand schools. This program is the only threat assessment model listed in the National Registry of Evidence-based Programs and Practices. A randomized controlled study of the Virginia Guidelines showed a 65 percent reduction in long-term suspensions, an 87 percent reduction in alternative school placements, nearly a 400 percent increase in the use of counseling, and a 250 percent increase in parental involvement (Cornell, 2013).

Conclusion

Lee Thompson Young was 29 years old, and by all outward appearances would seem to be on top of the TV world. He burst onto the scene at the age of 14 as the star of the Disney series *The Famous Jett Jackson*. His latest role cast him in a lead role in the show *Rizzoli & Isles*, a popular television show. By all rights, he was on top of the TV world, and had a bright future. Yet on Monday, August 19, 2003, he turned a gun on himself and snuffed out a promising career in an instant (Andreeva, 2013).

When one of the coauthors was a freshman in college, he woke up one morning to the news that one of his friends who was still in high school had died at a party. The party had gone into the early hours of the morning, and the other teens at the house awoke hours later to find their friend floating in a swimming pool. According to the other teens, he had been talking about huffing the night before and they believed he had drowned because he had been too disoriented to save himself from the relatively shallow pool. Tragedies like this always bring up the question: why did this happen seemingly without warning?

People who are going to commit violence against themselves, just like those who plan to harm others, usually exhibit at least some warning signs. In these two tragic cases where young people took their own lives—whether on purpose or by accident—there were undoubtedly some types of warning signs that were overlooked, ignored, or misunderstood by bystanders. In the case of the drowning, the young man's death probably would have been prevented if his friends had cued in on the warning signs. These signs included his increasing drug use combined with his hanging out at a house where stories of parties where sex and drug use with limited adult supervision were popular items of gossip among their group of friends. Learning to properly identify these signs could save lives from a violent attack but in many cases might save someone from his or her own actions. These signs can be used to classify the type of violence that may occur, as well as the proximity in time of the violence. These signs apply regardless of the age of the person, although the actual types of signs may vary.

Watch for the signs that a person is progressing along the continuum of violence, or for expressions of the seven survival signs that de Becker outlines. Practice identifying these techniques in others, and learn to trust your instincts when they tell you that a person may pose some risk for you.

This is even more important with children, since noticing the early warning signs is an opportunity for adults to intercede and provide help for the child, not to put them away in a hole somewhere. Learn the signs, and know what to do if you notice them.

Key Points in Chapter Five

- The continuum of violence is a path of escalation from low to high: intimidation, escalation, and further escalation. At the same time, people do not always proceed along this continuum in a direct line.
- Look for a change in normal behavior, with clusters of concerning behaviors.
- If someone's behavior bothers you, consider why it bothers you, and bring it to the attention of someone who can do something about it.
- One of the best survival skills we can develop is the ability to know when we are a potential target.

BIBLIOGRAPHY

Andreeva, N. (2013). UPDATE: "Rizzoli & Isles" stops production following Lee Thompson Young's death. *Deadline Hollywood*. Retrieved from *http://www. deadline.com/2013/08/r-i-p-lee-thompson-young/*

de Becker, G. (1997). *The gift of fear and other survival signals that protect us from violence*. New York: Dell Publishing.

Cornell, D. (2013), Threat assessment in Virginia schools. Presented at the 2013 Virginia School & Campus Safety Training Forum, State D.A.R.E. and NASSLEO Conference in Hampton, Virginia on August 7.

Dorn, M., and C. Dorn. (2008). *Warning signs of destructive youth behaviors and positive intervention action steps*. Macon, GA: Safe Havens International.

Kasindorf, M. (2006). Woman kills 5, self at postal plant. *USA Today*. Retrieved from *http://usatoday30.usatoday.com/news/nation/2006-01-31-postal-shooting_x.htm*

Postal killer believed she was target of a plot. (2006). Crime and Courts on NBCNews.com. Retrieved from *http://www.nbcnews.com/id/11167920/#. Ud3v_lOvt7Y*

Postal shooter's bizarre behavior. (2009). CBS News. Retrieved from *http://www.cbsnews.com/2100-201_162-1272077.html?pageNum=1*

Holmes, R., and S. Holmes. (2001). *Mass murder in the United States.* Upper Saddle River, NJ: Prentice Hall.

Holmes, R., and S. Holmes. (1998). *Serial murder* (2nd ed.). Thousand Oaks, CA: Sage Publications.

Skipp, C. (2010). Inside the minds of family annihilators. Retrieved from *http://www.thedailybeast.com/newsweek/2010/02/10/inside-the-minds-of-family-annihilators.html*

Things you should know about sexual offending. (2013). Retrieved July 26, 2013, from *http://sor.state.co.us/?SOR=home.youshouldknow*

Walker, J. (2012). Are mass shootings becoming more common in the United States? *Reason.com.* Retrieved from *http://reason.com/blog/2012/12/17/are-mass-shootings-becoming-more-common*

CHAPTER SIX

PREPARING YOUR SPACE

Or how minor adjustments in your work area can save your life.

The school registrar looked up as the woman entered the office. Her legs had metal braces and her hair was streaked with gray. She could be anyone's grandmother. She seemed irritated but in control of her emotions until the registrar told her that her grandchild lived outside of the school district and could no longer be enrolled at the school without paying out-of-county tuition.

In response, the woman went to the office door and locked it with the thumb lock, then turned back to the secretary's desk. She approached, picked up a wooden nameplate from the counter, and began to repeatedly beat the school employee with it. When the registrar tried to pick up the phone to call for help, the attacker ripped the phone off the wall and began to hit her over the head with it.

After the victim had been taken to the hospital, two school district police officers obtained a warrant for her arrest and headed to the nearby rural county where she lived. They met a deputy sheriff at the county line, where he informed the two officers that the suspect was already on probation for auto theft. Given the nature of the suspect, they might need backup. The two school officers were in disbelief. Surely the deputy wasn't scared of a grandmother with metal braces on both legs?

The suspect proved the deputy correct by retreating into a bedroom and putting up a fight that made the officers earn their salary that day. By the time they finally handcuffed her, she had destroyed the bedroom, and the three officers looked like they had just broken up a bar fight.

Once she was cuffed, the woman prepared herself for one final escape attempt. Gasping and moaning, she cried, "My chest hurts!" She was transported to the hospital by ambulance before being taken to jail, wasting thousands of taxpayer dollars. The aggressor was experienced enough with the criminal justice system to know how to create additional time and expenses for the department by faking a heart attack as she had done several times before.

Some of the most violent people also look the least threatening. Leaving weapons like a pair of scissors, a letter opener, or even a large and heavy nameplate on your desk can be a terrible mistake if the wrong person shows up at your office one day.

In this chapter, we will introduce a number of simple, yet effective, techniques you can use to help reduce the risk of being harmed. Police officers are trained to make it a habit not to stand in front of a door when they knock on someone's door, an experienced pilot will make a habit out of checking and double-checking critical instruments and systems before each takeoff. As you read this book, you will probably think of your own methods for increasing your day-to-day safety at home, at work, and elsewhere.

CPTED—Powerful Deterrence and Peace of Mind

Crime prevention through environmental design (CPTED) is a simple, effective crime prevention methodology that has been successfully applied for some four decades. It has been shown to be an effective crime deterrent in settings where ordinary people go about their regular daily patterns, such as schools, retail establishments, offices, housing complexes, and public transportation. These simple concepts have even been used to reduce the number of stabbings of inmates in Israeli prisons. These measures have also made these same places more comfortable, though the implementation of CPTED is often too subtle for the untrained eye to notice.

As with security cameras, metal detectors, and armed security personnel, CPTED cannot make crime and violence disappear on its own. Only when combined with other protective measures can

CPTED reliably reduce violence. Unlike many popular security approaches, CPTED has been proven to be effective through decades of research. This chapter will focus on providing a layperson's summary of this proven approach.

Natural Surveillance

Simply put, natural surveillance is the ability to see and hear others without the assistance of technology. The idea behind natural surveillance is that criminals are sometimes afraid of being seen and reported while they are in the act. Persons planning a sexual assault, robbery, or a mass casualty attack will often modify their behavior when they know they are being watched.

Unfortunately, many people are not aware of the benefits of natural surveillance. This is particularly true when we are surrounded by security technology, especially security cameras. In fact, people sometimes rely on cameras for their safety so much as to dismiss the benefits of other factors—like natural surveillance. They are not aware that criminals are often more afraid of being seen by somebody through a window than of being recorded by a camera on the wall. After all, a person can call the police, but a camera usually cannot. More often than not, there is nobody watching a security camera in real time.

People often have a false sense of security when there are cameras, assuming that cameras are installed to deter crime in real time. They do not know that cameras are usually more effective in helping investigate a crime than preventing it. As one of many cases that illustrate this, the killers at Columbine High School were obviously not deterred by the school's surveillance system. We are even familiar with one school shooting where a middle school student looked directly at a security camera and nodded before he shot another student.

A good way to remember the power of natural surveillance is to remember to look for ways to increase opportunities for people to be able to see and to be seen. Although there are some exceptions, good natural surveillance can disrupt an aggressor's plans. One example is tipping window shades so that people from outside assume they can be seen from inside. And while it may seem counterintuitive to many people, covering windows in your residence, office, school, or other setting in a way that prevents you from seeing outside can actually increase danger by reducing the chances that an imminent act of violence will be detected and stopped or mitigated.

Another way to increase natural surveillance is to align parking spaces so that occupants of a building can see between cars when looking out the window. Trimming shrubbery or tree limbs to minimize hiding spaces at a private residence, moving a vending machine that creates a visual barrier, and making a host of similar simple changes can also increase visibility. Positioning playground equipment in your yard in a location that allows better visibility not only will help prevent crime but can also allow you to see your children more clearly from inside the house so you can respond quickly if they injure themselves or have a medical emergency.

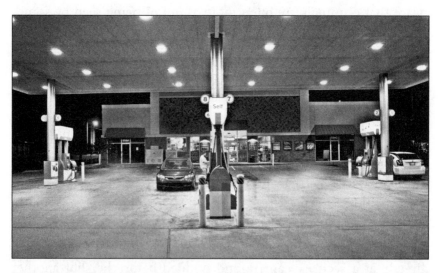

Natural surveillance: Designing a space with natural surveillance in mind can pay great dividends in reduced security technology costs and enhanced prevention. This gas station is designed so that it is easy for cashiers and customers to see between each car and gas pump, reducing the chances of illicit activity in parking areas without the need for additional security cameras.
Photo: Rachel Wilson

Natural surveillance also includes the ability to hear. For example, a woman is less likely to be sexually assaulted and students are less likely to be bullied in a restroom that has a doorless entryway because others are more likely to hear the attack and summon assistance (Atlas, 2013). You have probably noticed these types of restrooms in airports, schools, and public buildings. By using an entryway that channels people around corners instead of relying on doors, these restrooms are generally safer than traditional restrooms. For this reason, architects, security directors, and others who are well versed on CPTED often use these designs.

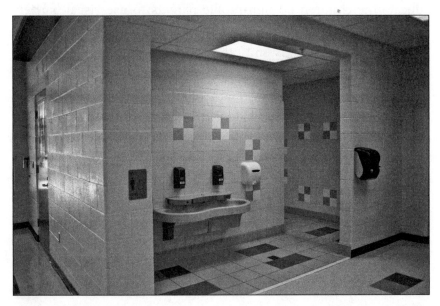

Open-door bathroom designs: This restroom in a Georgia school uses a design that is proven to be safer, because people outside the restroom can hear an assault, bullying, or other forms of aggression. This design also significantly reduces construction and maintenance costs.
Photo: Rachel Wilson

Of course there are situations where increased visibility can increase risk. A curbside window revealing a room filled with computers can increase the risk of burglary. Exposing a person who is at high risk for violent attack to public view can increase the risk of an attack. For example, it might not be a good idea for a public official at risk of assassination to be clearly visible through a large front window.

Schools also sometimes require modified approaches to increased natural surveillance. For example, when Amanda Mueller, who was the granddaughter of the founder of the Mueller Pasta Company, was nine years old, she was abducted from her independent school in Naples, Florida. Her kidnappers hid her in a refrigerator box in the woods and demanded $1.5 million in ransom money for her safe return. She was found safe four days later and her four abductors were arrested. (Girl survives, 1986). We often advise schools that educate the children of high-profile parents to use visual barriers or walls to make it more difficult for an aggressor to conduct surveillance of playgrounds and other open areas when planning an attack or abduction. At the same time, most criminals prefer areas that are more private, rather than open to public observation. This risk is often mitigated by the addition of armed bodyguards when high-profile targets or property are present as in the case in some independent schools.

When good natural surveillance is combined with preventive measures like access control, security personnel, logically applied camera surveillance, and other security concepts, the risks of crime and violence can be reduced even further.

Natural Access Control

The next CPTED concept that can help you reduce your personal risk of violence is natural access control. Even though there can definitely be an advantage to having physical access control technology like door buzzers with an intercom in a business or apartment building, natural access control takes advantage of the design of a building or area itself. The best example is limiting the number of access points to an area so that visitors encounter natural surveillance by people who have a stake in security. Natural access control can also help create a more open and friendly environment by improving access control and customer service for legitimate users of an area.

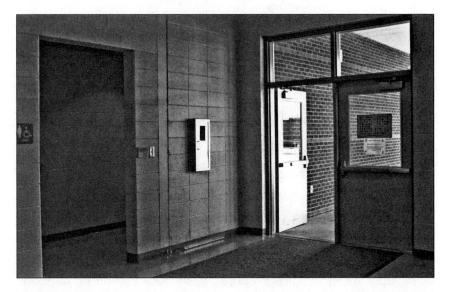

Natural access control: This photo shows a gap in natural access control—a propped exterior door—that could make it easier to sneak into an area to carry out an attack or to commit thefts.
Photo: Rachel Wilson

For example, placing a kiosk with a receptionist in the lobby of a high-rise office building can make it more difficult for an aggressor to enter the building to kill his ex-wife on the fifth floor without being seen. In another common example, we often work with architects to design school entryways that require visitors to enter through the main office. By using design features that channel visitors into the main office before they can enter the rest of the school, it becomes far more difficult for a noncustodial parent to sneak by the front office to abduct his or her child from a classroom. These design features also make it easier for legitimate users to find the front office. Though this approach alone may not stop a determined and armed aggressor, natural access control has proven to be effective at reducing the risk of many types of crimes, including some acts of armed aggression.

Natural access control often involves the physical design features of a building or an outdoor area, but simple practices like locking a door can also help. It is not unusual for several unlocked doors to lead to an administrative office suite. By minimizing the number of unlocked doors leading to an area, we can channel visitors through a doorway where employees can easily observe them, reducing the chances that an attacker will be able to surprise a victim.

Stake Your Claim with Territoriality

In CPTED, territoriality means creating a sense of ownership. This gives people a stake and a direct interest in the security of the facility because we tend to protect what we perceive as our own. Positive territoriality creates an environment where people are more likely to become involved in the safety and well-being of the community as a whole. For example, when people feel connected to a physical place, they are more apt to report a suspicious person or someone committing a crime.

This can be accomplished in many ways, including installing murals, personal artwork, landscaping, and in some cases technology like flat screen televisions in common areas. The way we create positive territoriality can depend on context.

One way of explaining the concept of territoriality is to look at a concept from the opposite end of the spectrum. The broken window theory is a concept that holds that the more damage and vandalism there is in an area, the more crime there will be. A study by the Stanford psychologist Philip Zimbardo showed that when a car has severe body damage it is more likely to be vandalized and picked apart by thieves (Wilson and Kelling, 1982). The logical response to this is the concept of territoriality, which promotes positive behavior and discourages illicit activity by setting a distinct tone and set of informal rules based on the connection between the building and its occupants.

There are usually simple and inexpensive ways to increase positive territoriality for any setting. Many people have difficulty seeing the connection between murals and security, but this connection is very well documented by research (Taylor, 2002). Coauthor Michael Dorn saw this technique in application while he was in Israel for training on antiterrorism as part of an international law enforcement exchange program operated by Georgia State University. During his visit, he toured two Israeli prisons. While visiting a women's prison, he was puzzled to see a number of inmates painting a very large mural of Russian Orthodox churches in a large room. As it turns out, this simple detail was part of a larger approach that has proven to be very effective.

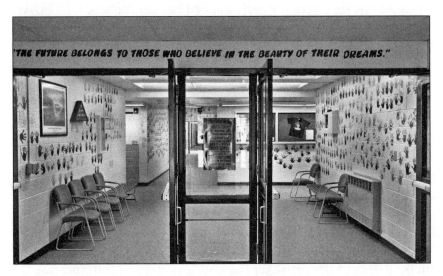

Territoriality: Improving the connection between people and the physical place is proven to reduce the risk of crime and the fear of crime as well. This hallway at an elementary school in Farmington, New Mexico, is an excellent example of low-cost integrated territoriality created through color schemes, positive decor, student artwork, and materials donated by local vendors.
Photo: Chris Dorn

An Israeli prison official explained that inmates in Israeli prisons are allowed to have knives and forks in their cells. Israeli inmates will rarely attack a correctional officer because they can lose their conjugal visits and annual 30-day furloughs, but they do sometimes attack fellow inmates with knives. The official commented that the assault rate in prisons where the inmates had been allowed to paint murals had dropped significantly. Dorn learned that many of the inmates in this particular prison were originally from Eastern Europe.

The use of positive territoriality can also help take the edge off of other security measures like security cameras and metal detectors. We often provide training and keynote presentations for architects, school superintendents, law enforcement personnel, homeland security professionals, and other practitioners in ways to dramatically increase physical security in schools and other settings without creating a prison-like environment.

Buildings that have properly applied the concepts of CPTED are generally more secure, more inviting, and promote more connectivity between people. The key concept of CPTED is to make it more comfortable for the legitimate user to occupy a space while decreasing the comfort level of a trespasser or other violator. This has been particularly effective in schools and other organizations, but it can also be applied by individuals at home and sometimes in other locations as well.

Target Identifiers

Some design features and practices can increase danger. *Target identifiers* are features that are potentially dangerous because they make it easier for an attacker to locate a victim and thus increase the chances of a successful attack. Target identifiers take many forms, most commonly either a reserved parking space or office that is marked by name. Schools also commonly place artwork or other signage outside each classroom that identifies the classroom occupants by name and sometimes even with photos of students. While these types of signs provide benefit for the occupant, they can make it easier for an aggressor to identify a victim. The name of a woman on her classroom or office doorway can help an abusive ex-husband find his target, and a row of cute photos of students alongside a classroom might literally be a menu for a child predator to choose his next victim from.

For example, a Wisconsin elementary school student was located and abducted from his classroom after his father—who did not have custody rights—found a way to defeat the school's access control.

Once inside the building, he walked down the halls until he found his child's teacher's name on the classroom door. He then forcefully abducted the child and removed him from the school. In other cases, teachers themselves have been attacked after an aggressor located their classroom in this manner.

We do advocate student artwork being used to improve the connection between students and their schools; however, even though photos of students and staff members are also great ways to improve the school décor, these should be used in consideration with this risk. A more appropriate practice would be to post student artwork or positive photos of students and staff members in common areas of the school so that they cannot be used to locate the individual.

In the example of reserved parking or offices, we call signs that say such things as "Reserved for Director of Human Resources"—or "Reserved for Mr. Johnson"—"shoot me" signs because they can and have been used by aggressors to locate and attack a victim or to simply vandalize the victim's car. The murder of a teacher who worked at one of the nation's most respected independent schools is a good example. After a bitter divorce, a man relentlessly hunted his ex-wife, who was a teacher. She had been hiding from him by living in different hotels, renting different cars, and varying her daily habits.

After she was murdered, a detective called the school's security director and informed him that the killer had confessed that he first tried to find and kill her at school, since he knew he could easily find her there. At the time they had been together, the man had noticed that the school marked each teacher's parking space with the teacher's name as a perk for staff members. When the security director was hired, he had advised the headmaster how dangerous this practice was, and the parking spaces were all repainted with a simple number. Because of this change, the killer in this case was unable to identify her parking space, and he was unwilling to go through the school's careful visitor screening process, as he might be detected and stopped. Though violators often do not fear incarceration or in some instances death, they often fear failure of their attack plan (Grossman, 2008).

Unfortunately, the teacher had not informed the security director of the school, whose team of superb security officers very well might have been able to save her life if she had sought their assistance. In the end, her efforts to avoid her ex-husband's vengeance proved fruitless because he was able to kill her in another setting. His actions were, however, delayed so that the children were spared the trauma of seeing one of their teachers murdered in broad daylight in the school parking lot.

This tragic incident demonstrates the benefits of eliminating target identifiers at a workplace to make it more difficult for an aggressor to locate a victim. Simply changing signage to read "Reserved" can make it much harder for an aggressor to find and attack a victim by staking out a particular car. If spaces need to be reserved for specific individuals, generic numbering is a better option that can also deter a trespasser from parking in areas other than assigned visitor parking. Channeling visitors to appropriate parking spaces in turn enhances the natural surveillance of the facility if these parking areas are visible to building occupants.

There can be other benefits from neutralizing target identifiers. For example, one of our clients was faced with a particularly challenging media situation, and the top executive for the organization exited out of a back door to avoid a barrage of reporters after a controversial meeting. As he reached his car, he found a full television crew set up next to his car, which was parked in a space marked with his title.

Another form of target identifier can be our clothing or other physical signs that indicate we are vulnerable. Wearing casual clothing and carrying a guide map and a large camera could indicate to potential thieves that you are a tourist and an easy target. Likewise, wearing a lanyard and name badge while wandering around near your conference hotel would indicate to a criminal that you are in town on business and that you are at a disadvantage when it comes to situational awareness because you are probably unfamiliar with the area and distracted by work. The aggressor could also reasonably assume that you could be carrying valuables like cash, a cell phone, rental car keys, and a laptop.

Similarly, making it too easy for an aggressor to wander into an office building and find a potential victim through building signage can dramatically reduce the effectiveness of building security should the aggressor find a way to breach primary access control systems. As described in Chapter Three, we have regularly been able to defeat a wide array of security technologies because a single person does something as simple as propping a door open with a rock. This makes a layered approach to security important.

Diagrams that show where specific offices are in an office building rather than simply indicating where an office suite is located are another common targeting identifier. For example, if someone wants to locate and kill an attorney after a nasty divorce, listing the exact location of the individual office on a diagram in the lobby can help an aggressor carry out an attack, as opposed to a more general map that only shows where the office suite for the firm is located.

Entrapment

As with target identifiers, entrapment increases the chances of a successful act of violence. *Entrapment* can be avoided—through careful consideration of the layout of an office. Furniture should be arranged in such a way so that an aggressor cannot trap someone inside the office or other workspace. The attack described at the beginning of this chapter is a good example. Because of the office layout, the secretary had only one escape route from her desk, and it was blocked by her aggressive sixty-five-year-old female visitor.

In another example, an angry and imposing man who was more than six feet tall visited a five-foot tall assistant principal. Due to the position of her desk, the assistant principal was trapped behind her desk while the aggressor yelled, screamed, and cursed at her. He simply stood in her only avenue of escape. Terrified from the experience, she now keeps a claw hammer under her desk. "This is not a weapon," she maintains, "It is a tool to fix broken parents!" Though we do not advocate that you keep a claw hammer under your desk or attack agitated customers, we do suggest you evaluate your workspace to see if there are ways you can reduce the chances that an aggressive person could trap you.

Ask anyone who has been in this type of situation, and the person will tell you that it leaves a deep and lasting impression. In fact, the story above is one of the most common examples of school violence that we run across. It is not uncommon to hear stories like this one from the schools we work with. One of our clients related the story of a staff member who was trapped behind her desk and then beaten so badly by an outraged student that she later died from her injuries after being hospitalized for several years. Even though there will often be restrictions created by the design of the facility itself, it is a good idea to look for ways to create multiple pathways and escape routes whenever possible. Sometimes this may only require that you move a desk a foot or two. In some cases, an entire office may need to be rearranged; in other instances, a significant alteration of the office layout may be required and might be a reasonable adjustment. For example, if your work requires you to regularly interact with angry people, it is more likely that you will someday be physically attacked, making such adjustments worth the time and expense. In other cases where there is a lower risk of physical violence, a more cost-effective option may be to make it a habit to have all meetings in a conference room or other area where an aggressor will not trap you and there are more bystanders to call for help in the event of violence.

The Presence of Improvised Weapons

The presence of items that can easily be seized and used as a weapon in an office area can also increase the risk of violence. This is how the aggressive grandmother in our example was able to instantly find a weapon to attack the secretary—in this case a large wooden nameplate on the counter.

Even though many people fear guns and knives the most, experienced police officers know that a surprising number of people are seriously injured and killed by improvised weapons each year. People are killed with baseball bats, claw hammers, screwdrivers, wrenches, tire irons, scissors, and an astounding variety of blunt and sharp objects. Many states have laws that create extra penalties for criminals who use guns or specific types of knives. Though valuable, laws prohibiting the possession of a firearm by a convicted felon can also influence the decision to select alternate forms of deadly weapons.

In many instances, a person who is angry, intoxicated, or dangerously mentally ill might simply pick up an object and use it as a weapon. As we discussed in the last chapter, even though people in these three categories are not always violent, they make up a large percentage of violent offenders. If you have a job that makes it necessary for you to periodically interact with people who are in one or more of these conditions on a regular basis, you should consider making it a habit not to have things in plain view in your work area that could be easily picked up and used to hurt you. In addition to the more common items listed above, we have also found a variety of souvenirs in work areas like spears, swords, baseball bats, and other objects that can easily be used to attack a staff member.

In one case in which one of the coauthors worked as a police officer, an intruder who was high on street drugs attacked a high school principal in his office with a machete. The principal had kept the machete propped in a corner of a bookcase behind his desk as a keepsake. Were it not for the amazingly fast reactions of a school district police officer, the man might have succeeded in trying to decapitate the principal with his own machete. The principal had laughed if off when school police had warned him about having the machete in his office, but he never left anything so dangerous in his office again.

Safe Rooms

One simple but powerful concept to help you address the risk of violence in your personal area is the establishment of one or more safe rooms. While high-risk facilities or persons might justify something more elaborate, this can often be as simple as making minor modifications to one or more existing rooms in a structure. For example, for many years, we have shown our school clients how to find ways to create a rapidly lockable space in office areas, cafeterias, media centers, and other key areas of a school or support facility that are not easily secured.

At home, a safe room can be any room that you can quickly retreat into and lock yourself inside to avoid violence or create more challenges for an attacker to get to you to carry out an act of violence. However, many interior doors and locks lack the strength to prevent a determined aggressor from forcing his way into a room. In these cases, you may consider installing a stronger door and/or locking system with the understanding that this approach will only delay an attacker for a short period of time.

The concept of safe rooms not only requires us to locate a place to hide but also to consider the speed at which you can lock a door in a crisis. This could be one of the most important skills you will ever need to apply. For example, the difference between life and death for students in an elementary school can depend on something as simple as how fast a teacher can lock a single door when an armed intruder is in the school. One teacher taking forty-five seconds to find a key, insert it in a lock, and secure the door can be twenty-five seconds too late to prevent the deaths of multiple children. When choosing safe rooms in your house, verify not only that the door locks are in working condition but that their design also allows you to quickly lock them from the inside.

Besides locking mechanisms, communication systems in a safe room are also important to consider. By thinking about wiring in an extension to the school intercom system, keeping a clear path, and selecting a room with a telephone, school office staff who are confronted with an aggressor can quickly retreat to this room, lock the door, announce a lockdown for the rest of the school, and call 911. Many schools have prepared their employees to perform all of these functions in 10–15 seconds by installing duress buttons in their safe rooms and encouraging regular practice. If we contrast this approach with trying to order a lockdown and call the police while trying to fight off an armed aggressor, it is easy to see how important it can be to think about safe rooms in your home or place of work. This is especially critical in K–12 schools where the safety of hundreds or even thousands of staff and students can be at stake. If a safe room requires a radio or cell phone to communicate with the outside world, these devices should be tested periodically in that location. If your safe room is in an office vault or in the basement of your home, will you be able to get a cell signal through the increased thickness of walls or ceilings?

The Benefits of Darkness

While we tend to think of darkness as dangerous, this is not always the case. For example, some organizations have reduced the frequency of crimes like burglary, arson, and vandalism by using lights-out policies when facilities are not in use. This is because criminals in a dark building are forced to use flashlights or some other form of illumination to see what they are doing, increasing the chances that a security patrol or passerby will report their activity. The Watergate scene in the film *Forrest Gump* is a good illustration of this concept in a dramatized form. When Gump sees men using flashlights in an adjacent office building, he inadvertently causes the men to be caught because he reports behavior that he judged to be out of the ordinary. Though this is a fictional account, it is representative of how many criminals have been caught in actual incidents.

In a real-life example, a burglar was apprehended by a Bibb County school district police officer who found a trail of candle wax on the floor of a school where a silent alarm had been tripped. The trail of wax led to a girl's restroom, where the officer found the suspect standing on a toilet in the last stall, holding a knife and waiting to attack. The school's lights-out policy had forced the suspect to use a candle to see what he was doing. Armed with a semiautomatic pistol, a good flashlight, and good tactics, the officer was able to take the suspect into custody without anyone being hurt.

Brightness can also make people and property more visible and vulnerable. For example, if you arrive for work early in the morning and have to park in a parking space that is well lit, then you walk through a poorly lit area to enter the building, a criminal can see you and attack you while you have limited night vision. If you instead park in an area where you are not illuminated (preferably in an open area of the parking lot), you can make it harder for an aggressor to sneak up on you. By sweeping the parking area with your headlights set on high beam before you park, you can disrupt an aggressor's vision. You could go so far as to disable your car's interior light and slam the door twice to make it sound like you are not alone. A high-intensity flashlight can be an effective method to further disturb an aggressor's night vision. While each of these strategies has its limitations, you can see how lighting may or may not interfere with an aggressor's attack plan.

Similarly, lighting on the inside of your residence at night can help an aggressor more than you. Because you are much more familiar with the layout of your house, for example where furniture is located, an aggressor would need the light to navigate more than you do. Turning off the lights in your house forces an intruder to use a light or increases the chances that he will trip, alerting you to his presence.

There are many factors that must be considered, since a lights-out policy can indeed increase the risk of crime in some situations. For example, the lights-out approach could increase the danger of assault during an evening meeting at an office complex parking lot. The key is to understand that having a well-lit area does not always benefit the potential victim. Understanding lighting and how it can work for and against you can be a valuable asset in preventing crime or defending yourself during an attack.

Conclusion

Adjustments to our work setting can reduce risk. These adjustments are usually relatively simple enough to be developed into regular habits without a great deal of effort. Making a reasonable effort in these areas can have a truly profound effect on the chances that we will be attacked successfully. Most importantly, when considering the safety and security of your personal space, think beyond traditional technology-based security systems, and consider how the overall design, layout, and use of your space can be used to your advantage.

Key Points in Chapter Six

- Some of the most violent people also look the least threatening.
- Criminals are often more afraid of being seen by somebody through a window than of being recorded by a security camera.
- Remember to look for ways to increase opportunities for people to be able to see and be seen. Buildings that have properly applied the concepts of CPTED (crime prevention through environmental design) are generally more secure and more inviting and promote more connectivity between people.
- Natural access control can limit the number of access points to an area and help create a more open and friendly environment by improving access control and customer service for the legitimate users of an area.
- By minimizing the number of unlocked doors leading to an area, we can channel visitors through a doorway where they can be observed.
- With positive territoriality, people are more likely to become involved in the safety and well-being of the community as a whole because it promotes positive behavior and discourages illicit activity by setting a distinct tone.
- The more vandalism there is in an area, the greater the risk of crime there may be.

- *Target identifiers* make it easier for an attacker to locate a victim, increasing the chance of a successful attack. In a school, these might be the names of students near a classroom; for others, it might be wearing a conference badge or a tourist's attire while wandering around an unfamiliar town.
- Furniture should be arranged in such a way so that an aggressor cannot trap you inside your office or other workspace.
- A safe room can be any room that you can quickly retreat into and lock yourself inside to avoid violence or create more challenges for an attacker to get to you.

BIBLIOGRAPHY

Atlas, R. I. (2013). *21st Century security and CPTED: Designing for critical infrastructure protection and crime prevention* (2nd ed.). Boca Raton, FL: CRC Press.

Girl survives kidnapping in box. (1986, September 28). *Lawrence Journal-World.* Retrieved from *http://news.google.com/newspapers?id=38IxAAAAIBAJ&sjid= teUFAAAAIBAJ&pg=4960%2C5022515*

Grossman, D. (2008). The bulletproof mind: Prevailing in violent encounters . . . and after [DVD]. Delta Media.

Taylor, R. B. (2002). Crime prevention through environmental design (CPTED): Yes, no, maybe, unknowable, and all of the above. In R. B. Bechtel (Ed.), *Handbook of environmental psychology* (pp. 413–426). New York: John Wiley.

Wilson, J., and G. Kelling. (1982). Broken windows; The police and neighborhood safety. Retrieved from *http://www.manhattan-institute.org/pdf/ _atlantic_monthly-broken_windows.pdf*

CHAPTER SEVEN

THE IMPORTANCE OF PREPARING PROPERLY

Or how you can use simple drills to learn how to live.

On a December morning in 1958, an elementary school child struck a match in the basement of the Our Lady of the Angels Catholic School (OLA) in Chicago. He had received a hall pass but had instead made his way into the unlocked boiler room where he found some trash that he used to start a small fire underneath a wooden staircase. It turned into a massive blaze that killed 92 students and 3 teachers, making this the most deadly attack to date at an American school. The true cause of the fire was only uncovered when a polygraph examiner obtained a confession from the boy, who gave a chilling explanation of why he had set the deadly fire three years before:

> "Why did you set the fire?" Mr. Reid asked. The boy's voice turned bitter: "Because of my teachers," he said. "I hated my teachers and my principal. They always were threatening me. They always wanted to expel me from school." (Brendtro, 2005)

The OLA fire is well known among emergency response workers and had a lasting effect on fire codes and practices. There are a number of lessons that are applicable today in dangerous situations where life or death decisions must be made. While locking the boiler room door or more closely supervising students may have prevented the incident, it is likely that small modifications in the school's fire drills would have allowed every one of these 95 people to stay alive. Like many schools today, there was a simple but common flaw in how the school conducted its nine fire drills every year.

At OLA, the headmaster activated the alarm during each fire drill. Staff and students filed out of the building in a prompt and orderly fashion. Fire drills were taken very seriously, and students and staff could normally clear the building in less than three minutes. The problem in this methodology is that the principal of a school is not always the first person to identify a crisis like an active shooter or a fire—just like the fire at OLA.

In her book *The Fire That Will Not Die*, Michele McBride, an OLA survivor who was badly burned before jumping out of a third story window to escape, describes how her teacher ordered her and the other students to wait and pray the Rosary instead of evacuating. According to McBride, the nun told the whole class that they could not evacuate because the head of school had not yet sounded the fire alarm. While this reaction may seem bizarre, it occurred in more than one classroom that day (McBride, 2004). This happened because the teachers did exactly what they had practiced: they evacuated when the fire alarm sounded—not when the fire was spotted or when a teacher saw smoke filling a stairwell but when someone else pulled the alarm.

You may not be able to understand this reaction while calmly sitting and reading this book. The employees at OLA were experiencing the very real stress reactions of a life and death situation. Under extreme stress, people often do exactly what they have practiced without separating the action steps they should take from the instructions and other extraneous information from their drills and training. We know this because people under stress have acted in bizarre ways. They in fact often do things that defy logic. While fire drills are obviously not intended to condition teachers to remain in a burning building until, and only until, the fire alarm has sounded, this is exactly what happened at OLA.

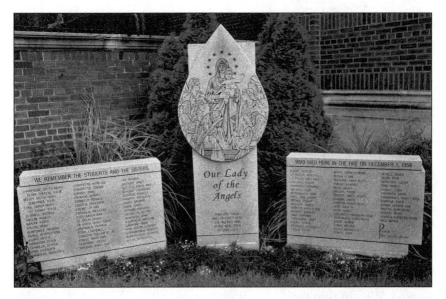

OLA: The most lethal attack at an American school was an arson fire set by a student at the Our Lady of Angels Sacred Hearts School in 1958. The school's principal pulled the fire alarm for all monthly fire drills, which inadvertently conditioned some staff members to wait to evacuate until the alarm was sounded. This contributed to the deaths of 95 staff and students.
Photo: Charles Fleming

One of the main components of a drill is the physical memory and experience of performing life-saving action steps, like getting out of the building quickly and safely. In a crisis, we are often forced to rely on physical memory rather than logical thought processes. This incident vividly illustrates how people in a crisis may do exactly what they practice in a drill, and why emergency plans and drills must take into account the effects of life and death stress on the human mind. As Grossman states: "We do not rise to the occasion, we sink to the level of our training" in a crisis (Dorn, 2012).

The Devastating Effects of Life and Death Stress on the Unprepared Mind

Let's look at how life and death stress can degrade the ability of the unprepared mind. The reactions of the educators at OLA are, at face value, shocking. Why would these dedicated and educated individuals allow themselves and children to die for the sake of following a procedure? We now know they were in effect inadvertently "drilled to death." Today we have research to help us understand why these individuals responded this way. We know that the human mind and body react in specific, predictable ways under life and death stress. When the heart rate accelerates considerably, the effects can be detrimental to our survival in certain ways, but these are actually evolved behaviors that are a response to threats that humans faced long ago.

For example, our bodies physiologically react in a way that helps improve the ability of our major muscle groups to help fight with more stamina and run faster.

According to Grossman, there is an optimal range at which we can operate under stress, between 115 and 145 beats per minute (bpm). Within that range our body sends help in the form of heightened physiological awareness and response, but as the stress level increases, the effects of this bodily response can begin to hinder our ability to respond. At this point, the body begins shutting down certain processes to focus efforts on the fight or flight response, so we lose more and more of our advanced cognitive and physical ability. Grossman states that the best way to overcome this challenge is through practice—for example, rehearsing the actions of dialing 911 on your cell phone or quickly locking or unlocking your door with your keys (Gladwell, 2005).

These are two areas where we commonly see stress reactions adversely affecting our response—for example, forgetting to press "send" when pressing 911 or fumbling with keys for a prolonged period of time when under extreme stress. In simulations in schools and other settings, we find that it can take some persons anywhere from 15 seconds to well over a minute to find their keys and either unlock a door to enter a safe area or lock a door to secure themselves from danger. This type of delay could be critical if you are faced with an impending threat like an attacker or severe weather.

As the heart rate approaches 175 bpm, we can expect to experience challenges like reduced cognitive processing abilities, auditory exclusion, and tunnel vision (Ripley, 2008). This means that we do not reason as effectively as normal, we may not hear certain sounds, and we may not see things that we need to see. As the heart rate climbs higher, we can expect to experience even more profound effects, like the irrational behavior exhibited by the nuns in 1958 (Grossman and Christensen, 2011). Some groups, like soldiers and law enforcement officers, are trained to counter the physical effects of crisis stress. At his private security firm, Gavin de Becker counters this with incredibly realistic training that involves trainees being shot with training rounds so they feel the real effects of stress. Through this process, he is able to reduce their heart rate during moments of intense pressure from around 145 bpm to 115 bpm. This allows trainees to better modulate their response and stay effective even under unexpected and dramatic situations (Gladwell, 2005).

Training can also help you overcome some of the low-level effects of crisis stress like trembling hands or hyperventilation. When you practice things like fire drills, safety briefings, or CPR, you are similarly training your body and mind to be ready to react fluidly while your decision-making processes are focused on processing information.

You should factor for these extreme stress effects when developing plans for an emergency. You should also consider the possibility that you or your family may not be able to perform certain tasks as easily when under extreme stress. Without taking this into consideration, there is a greater chance that your plans will fail during a real crisis. In the case of the 1958 school fire, the school did not consider the impact of extreme stress in its school crisis plan. In fairness, school officials in 1958 would not have been aware of these effects because much of the research in this field is fairly recent. They had little way of knowing how much crisis stress could affect our response to a life or death situation.

In our safety, security, and emergency preparedness assessments for schools, we perform one-on-one interviews with school staff to evaluate how school personnel would respond to an emergency. In these interviews, we run a series of crisis simulations using dynamic video scenarios that depict various crisis situations. Staff then have a chance to respond to verbal scenarios in the same way. Using scoring sheets, we are then able to tally the "fail rate" for critical action steps like activating the fire alarm, implementing a lockdown, sheltering for a tornado, calling 911, and responding to other life and death situations. Some of the responses to these interviews are truly astounding. Our clients are typically shocked at the actual reactions of their employees in contrast to what they expect them to do during a crisis.

It is important to understand that the level of stress during these simulations is a fraction of the stress that would result from a real crisis. These findings help us understand why there is often a delay of one to eight minutes before school employees make the decision to lock down during an actual school shooting. In some school shootings, a lockdown is never even announced (Alert system, 2005). This indicates that staff may wait or even forget to call a lockdown under stress. These failures have led some to the erroneous conclusion that the concept of lockdown is inherently flawed.

We must be careful not to confuse the failure of a concept with a failure in the application of the concept. Some have concluded that lockdowns are not effective because some victims have died in schools that have lockdown protocols on paper. They typically cite the Virginia Tech attack and the students who were killed in the library of Columbine High School as proof. However, the classrooms at Virginia Tech were not equipped with locks, and there were no faculty lockdown procedures. There had obviously not been any lockdown drills at the school. Similarly, the library at Columbine High School was never locked during the shooting in 1999. Abandoning the lockdown concept based on incidents like these is like saying that car door locks do not work because a thief entered an unlocked car and stole items. The failure is in the application of the locking mechanism and not the concept of locking doors.

As of this writing, we have not found or been provided with more than one example of an instance of lockdown concept failure in a

K–12 school. This is the Red Lake Reservation School shooting, which we will discuss later. Even this instance involved application failure because there was a secondary escape route that was not used in time. Keeping in mind that hundreds if not thousands of people have survived mass casualty shootings at schools without physical injury by using lockdowns, we urge caution if abandoning this approach is under consideration.

Proper Plans Promote Proper Preparedness

In order for you and your loved ones to be prepared to face emergencies, you need a plan. This can help you prepare to respond rapidly during an incident and will improve your ability to communicate with others and reunite afterwards.

Having an emergency plan is not enough—the plan needs to be technically sound and realistically practiced. This is true for families and any type of organization. One source of good information for developing family emergency plans is the U.S. Department of Homeland Security (Exercises, 2012). As we shall see, there are significant differences between appropriate planning for organizations and the way a family would develop a plan.

Use a Planning Process

There are different elements that can affect the quality of an emergency plan. The planning process itself provides a critical component of preparedness. To illustrate why the planning process is so important, it might be helpful to explain why organizations that skip this process often experience so many problems when a crisis occurs. For example, some organizations buy what is commonly referred to in the field of emergency management as a "plan in a can." These generic plans are not reliable because they are not developed based on local conditions.

For example, if you work in rural areas such as those found in parts of South Dakota, Montana, New York, Pennsylvania, and Texas, the first law enforcement personnel to arrive in a life and death situation may not arrive for 15 to 20 minutes after a call to 911. In some cases, response times are even slower. There are some regions of the country where officers may not arrive for more than an hour. Plans that might work in a suburb of Atlanta or Phoenix could fail miserably in these settings. In the same manner, plans that might work quite well in a community of 50,000 residents may not work so well in a large metropolitan area like Miami or Los Angeles.

Police training, tactics, and equipment also vary widely across the nation, even within individual states and regions. Local fire services, emergency medical services, and emergency management capabilities also vary widely. Although it is tempting to simply purchase an emergency plan, this generic approach is highly subject to failure and increased exposure to civil liability. Our expert witness work has shown us that the exposure to civil liability often increases significantly along with the risk of serious injury or death with this approach.

Perhaps an even more compelling reason to avoid using canned plans is that this approach circumvents the process of planning itself. The planning process occurs when an organization, be it a family, a small business, a school system, a synagogue, or a Fortune 500 company, identifies the challenges that may come up in an emergency situation. At almost every school emergency plan development meeting we have attended, an employee of the organization or a public safety official has identified at least one serious obstacle that needs to be addressed. Typically, planning team members will spot a number of significant challenges that must be addressed in order for the organization to be adequately prepared. There is a limited ability to develop a plan customized for these risks when emergency plans are simply purchased or copied rather than developed by an in-house team.

It is much better to find challenges and identify solutions in advance rather than to work them through in the middle of a crisis. Obviously, a mass casualty shooting is not the best time to find out that the lock on a classroom or a safe room does not work. There are many cases where these issues were not identified until after a crisis, resulting in serious injuries and death.

A shooting that took place at a school in Arkansas in 1998 serves as a stark example. In this incident, two youths activated the school's fire alarm system, then waited in the wooded area outside the school, opening fire on students and staff as they evacuated the school. Because the school had not planned, trained, and practiced what is known as a reverse evacuation, some school staff were not able to unlock exterior doors upon hearing the gunshots from the outside. This resulted in many students being trapped outside the school and exposed to more gunfire (Kifner, 1998). Five lives were taken and another ten innocent people were injured in this particular attack. More lives might have been saved if the victims had been prepared to return to the school immediately upon hearing gunfire.

While you may or may not be involved with the planning process for your place of work, learning, or worship, you will be involved if you decide to develop a plan for your family. In either case, taking the time to develop a plan can help you learn to react more effectively for any type of crisis.

Follow an All-Hazards Approach for a Sound Plan

Another element necessary for a sound plan is an all-hazards approach. This means that crisis plans should address a wide array of hazards rather than just those that we may think of first. For example, plans for an office park in Oklahoma that do not address hazardous materials incidents would be just as inadequate as if it did not include plans for a tornado. Tornadoes would be a specific concern for Oklahoma, but fire, hazardous materials incidents, and acts of violence can also occur in Oklahoma or any other state. This means a family emergency plan should cover not just violence but also natural disasters like a flood or a tornado and other man-made incidents like a serious car accident. One of the most common preparedness gaps we see is the pervasive tendency for people to focus intently on active shooter situations.

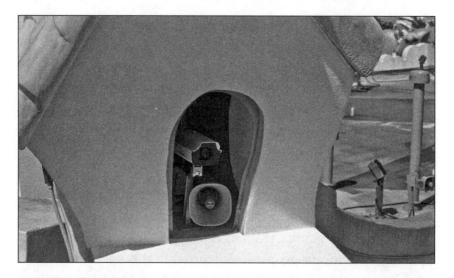

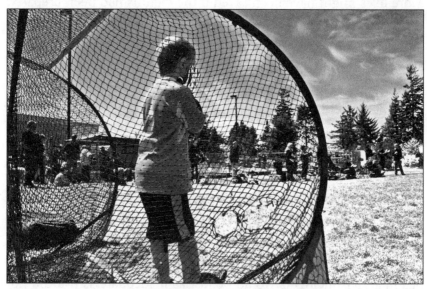

Places you frequent: Risk is present anywhere you live, play, study, shop, work, or worship. By taking ownership of your own safety and taking appropriate steps based on the all-hazards approach to risk reduction, you can reduce this risk. Even amusement parks need significant safety and security measures in place.
Photos: Rachel Wilson

Your family preparedness plan should also cover the places you frequent, like a movie theater, a shopping mall, or a park. When traveling to another region or country, you should take into account unique concerns and weather conditions specific to your new location. For example, when traveling to some coastal areas you should consider the threat of a tsunami, and an increased risk of crime or violence may be a factor when visiting major urban centers.

Consult with Your Local Emergency Management Agency

Whether you are developing a plan for your family or are on the planning team for an organization, you should consider seeking assistance from someone with an emergency management background. Crisis planning is not a predominant skill set for fire service and law enforcement officials. As a result, plans developed by people with a primary background in law enforcement are often "cop heavy" and do not address other hazards that are more present. This unbalanced focus on crime and violence usually results in plans with extensive information on active shooter situations and violence and limited information on other important types of hazards. Natural disasters often result in mass casualties, so ignore them at your own peril.

Emergency management officials are taught to think more broadly than any other public safety discipline. Although most emergency managers do come from another public safety field, they undergo specific training to help them understand the importance of the mindsets of the various disciplines they interact with. They also work to serve as a liaison for these agencies and help balance different viewpoints and sometimes conflicting approaches. Due to this unique role of serving as a hub rather than a stand-alone discipline, emergency managers tend to evaluate emergency preparedness approaches in a more holistic manner. For example, emergency managers often focus more on testing emergency preparedness measures that are relevant to any crisis rather than only one or two specific types of incident such as active shooter. Emergency managers will generally recommend that drills and exercises focus on crisis decision making and communications rather than on how a specific incident like a hostage situation will be resolved.

Sometimes operated through the local or state office of homeland security, fire department, or law enforcement organization, emergency management agencies can be an invaluable free resource. Because they are typically low-profile organizations or departments within a larger organization, emergency management professionals are often overlooked during the emergency planning process. Failing to obtain their assistance can result in reduced plan quality and, in some instances, increased exposure to civil liability. Most local and state emergency management agencies are not adequately staffed to provide intensive one-on-one assistance for a family developing a preparedness plan; nevertheless, they often will be able to provide resources that can be of help. There are some instances where they will work with groups of families who live in an area where there is a particular risk, like flash floods or chemical exposure.

Regardless of who helps develop plans, they should be tested, and the people who will implement them should practice their roles. Drills and exercises should be designed to allow practice in decision making. Of particular value are activities that drive home the need to be prepared, to adapt, and to think on the fly. With any plan, you should be prepared to take independent action and even deviate from it if following the plan as written would be more dangerous than adapting and taking a different course. We will explore specific ways this can be accomplished in the next section as we discuss the various types of drills and exercises organizations can use to improve survivability.

Drills—Turning Your Plans to Reality

In order to perform at high levels, you will need to practice your plans thoroughly. Relying on written plans that have not been tested is like learning how to jump out of an airplane by reading an instruction manual on the topic and attending a skydiving webinar. You might manage to survive if you have a good manual and study it carefully, but you will have much better odds of things going well if you test the concepts you have learned along the way with practical applications of what you have learned.

One of the important elements in conducting drills is that you should drill exactly the way you want to perform in reality. As illustrated in the OLA fire, school staff performed exactly the same steps as they had drilled. We call this effect "drilling to death" because people can be conditioned to die by improperly designed drills. This is how the powerful effects of crisis stress can cause a person to react in such a bizarre fashion during a real crisis.

There are a variety of types of drills and exercises that can dramatically improve emergency preparedness for an organization. Even though drills that allow physical practice are important, drills that offer all employees a chance to mentally simulate crisis decision making are among the most effective ways to address these gaps. The Federal Emergency Management Agency (FEMA) recommends that organizations use a progressive exercise program that includes drills along with orientation on the plan, tabletop exercises, functional exercises, and full-scale exercises. This type of progressive exercise program focuses primarily on decision making by leaders in various agencies. The primary opportunities for line-level staff to practice mental simulation and decision making lie within a specific subset of drills that we will discuss later.

We urge our clients to follow the progressive exercise approach advocated by FEMA. By utilizing a series of different types of drills and exercises over time, organizations can afford their employees an opportunity to practice while testing their plans, procedures, and equipment. The progressive exercise approach also allows organizations to practice working with one another and builds confidence and competency. For more information on the progressive exercise approach, FEMA offers a free independent study course on exercise design. For more about this course, visit *www.SafeHavens International.org.*

These types of drills and exercises have their limits. For example, law enforcement agencies routinely participate in exercises, but they also use a wide array of other training approaches to provide endless opportunities for independent life and death decision making. Even a robust drill and exercise program cannot give every participant the chance to make a wide range of critical decisions under time pressure. For example, in a full-scale active shooter exercise, there may be several hundred or more role players, but only a handful of those participants will make key decisions. Police agencies fill in these training gaps using mental simulation and other practices that allow officers to make decisions on their own. By combining mental simulation with the drill and exercise process, officers are given the chance to operate both individually and as a team in a major crisis event like an active shooter or hostage situation.

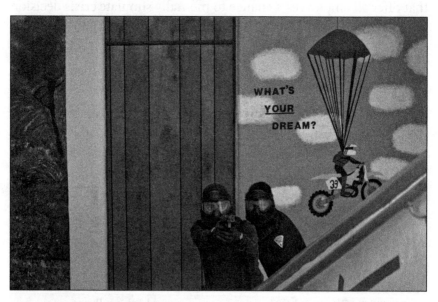

Police training exercise: Police officers in Farmington, New Mexico, hold an active shooter drill in a vacant school. These types of tactics were not widely used in the U.S. until after the deadly attack at Columbine High School in Colorado in 1999 but are now fairly advanced.
Photo: Rachel Wilson

Like a police agency, other organizations can easily and significantly improve their employees' level of preparedness with some simple modifications in existing emergency drills. Some years ago, coauthor Michael Dorn developed a concept that has become known as the "Dorn Drill." Dorn Drills change basic emergency drills—like fire drills—from a rote activity to an exercise in decision making and mental preparation. Using his work on after action reviews of school shootings along with the lessons learned from the OLA fire, he realized that school staff were still being inadvertently conditioned to wait for instructions from others during life and death emergencies. For example, in the 1958 OLA fire, all 95 deaths occurred because the fire alarm was not activated for approximately five minutes after the first teacher detected the fire. We have seen similar reactions in more recent mass casualty shootings and other catastrophic events.

The traditional approach to emergency drills is in direct opposition to the way most professionals in life and death fields prepare to operate in emergency situations. In contrast, Dorn Drills are in line with what we know from research on crisis stress, requiring that supervisors, managers, and executives empower employees to a high degree during a life or death emergency. This means that people in an organization should also be given a reasonable degree of guidance on what they should do in an emergency. This usually takes the form of crisis plans, training, and drills.

In his book *Streetlights and Shadows*, Dr. Gary Klein describes how he has found that although many high-stakes decision makers have written emergency procedures to guide them, they typically rely more on experience than written plans and checklists (Klein, 2009). For example, Klein describes how commercial and military pilots do not rely on emergency checklists for many of the life and death situations they encounter. U.S. Airways Captain Sully Sullenberger, who landed flight 1549 in the Hudson River with no fatalities or major injuries, said that he had checklists and charts to use during a crash landing, but "There wasn't time to do the math . . . I was quickly running through a host of facts and observations that I had filed away over the years, giving me a broad sense of how to make this decision—the most important one of my life" (Sullenberger, 2012).

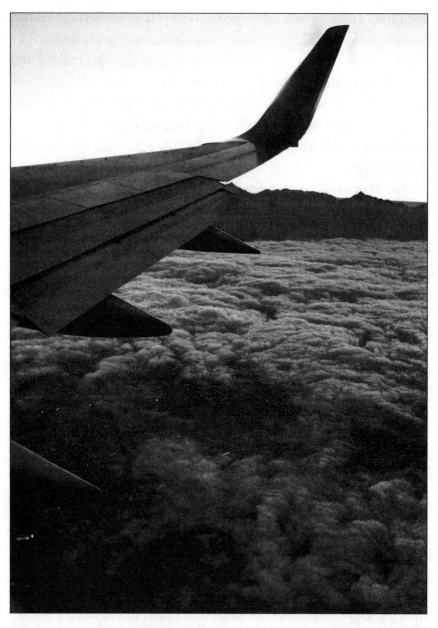

Hudson river plane crash: Examples like the landing of U.S. Airways flight 1549 on the Hudson River remind us that it is possible—and even statistically likely—that one will survive a plane crash. Paying attention to safety briefings and mentally simulating an emergency evacuation can significantly improve one's odds of survival in a crash.
Photo: Rachel Wilson

An airline pilot or police officer has the benefit of experiencing a large number of life and death situations to learn from over his or her career. For a business professional or an educator, this type of experience is not usually practical or desirable. We will focus on ways organizations can help their personnel practice in a cost- and time-efficient manner that is consistent with research, evaluation, and assessment. This approach raises a critical question: are the leaders of an organization confident in the ability of their staff—all staff—to take action to prevent death without overreacting?

To reduce the chances that these types of reactions will occur, Dorn Drills use a logical extension of the blocked access fire drill approach that has been in use for decades. In a blocked access fire drill, building occupants are required to seek alternate routes when signage or some other indicator simulates blocked emergency egress during the drill. This forces evacuees to think and act independently to find another way out of the facility. Likewise, a Dorn Drill elicits a response from line-level staff members who might be the first ones to discover danger. In a Dorn Drill, individual employees are prompted to begin a drill when a supervisor presents them with a verbal scenario rather than instructing them to take any specific action.

For example, instead of having a facilities worker activate the fire alarm to start a fire drill, a manager might approach an employee at his or her workstation and ask, "What would you do if you noticed that there was a black column of smoke coming from under that door and it was apparent that there was a fire behind the door?" Assuming a fairly typical set of emergency plan action steps for the organization, a proper response would sound something like this:

> I would tell everyone that there's a fire and that they need to evacuate. I would go out the back door and pull the fire alarm. I would then call the fire department on my cell phone and then I would call you [a supervisor] to tell you what happened.

If an appropriate response were given, the manager would tell the employee to perform the action steps. The fire department or alarm company should be notified of the drill in advance if the fire alarm system automatically notifies them. You should also check with 911 to see how they would like you to simulate the call to the dispatch center. In some areas, they will allow you to actually dial 911 after notifying them that you are about to conduct a drill. In large urban areas, the 911 center may request that you do not place a call for these types of drills. If this is the case, the call will need to be simulated in another way. For example, the employee can simulate the call with a desk phone that has been unplugged by the supervisor. An important point here is that any incorrect actions should be immediately corrected and the employee asked to perform them again the right way. Treat this as a learning process rather than a form of criticism. One way of approaching this would be to explain to the employee that you are learning something new as well. The purpose of this exercise is to create increased awareness and confidence, not a sense of inadequacy.

Many of the schools we work with use this method to initiate their fire, tornado, lockdown, and other drills. This approach to drills should only be used *after* proper procedures have been established, *after* all staff have been trained to implement them, and *after* employees have been told how these new types of drills will be conducted. For example, many schools lack an important emergency protocol known as a "room clear" procedure. Based on a protocol that the authors learned about from the Lincoln County School District in Newport, Oregon, this protocol can be used to clear students rapidly from a classroom, lunchroom, library, or gymnasium with a simple phrase (Dorn and Graves, 2010).

If a new procedure like this one is added, staff and students must be trained so that they understand expected action steps before a drill is held. Conducting drills in this manner for different types of emergency situations and asking different employees to make decisions makes it clear to all employees that they are not only authorized and empowered to take immediate life-saving action but also expected to do so. In the next chapter, we will show how a technique called mental simulation can be used to prepare more effectively and augment the use of Dorn Drills.

Conclusion

Like most people, you probably lead a very busy life. More than any other time in history, you are connected to countless people and sources of information. Television, radio, smartphones, e-mail, search engines, and an astounding array of social media allow us to interact with everyone from family and close friends to colleagues in far-off places like Qatar, Japan, and Argentina. Unlike your grandparents, you have a variety of 24-hour news channels to choose from, and even the local newspaper website can update you on breaking news within minutes. You spend more and more time commuting to and from work each day. If you have children, you likely spend a considerable amount of time taking them to and from the myriad of activities kids participate in these days. You may also be spending many hours each week caring for aging parents. With so much going on in your life, is it really practical for you to take the time needed to learn and internalize the survival skills described in this book?

Developing emergency plans, holding training sessions, and coordinating a progressive exercise program can be quite time and labor intensive for an organization; however, learning how to apply these concepts effectively can often be accomplished with relatively little time and energy on the individual level once plans have been developed. Some of the most effective techniques are those that take little time but happen at a higher frequency. In our experience, five to ten minutes a week of thoughtful activity will probably increase your ability to survive much more that the same amount of time spent during a single day each year (Dorn, 2012). Considering the permanency of serious injury and death, taking the time to prepare for emergencies is at least as logical as planning for your retirement. If you fail to plan for emergencies, you might not live long enough to enjoy the retirement you spend a large portion of your time and money planning for.

Shorter, more frequent, well-considered activities are often more effective at creating effective habits for one simple reason. This approach keeps your mind focused on emergency preparedness through repetition of regular application each day instead of only a few times a year. If you are able to combine both approaches, an even greater effect will usually be achieved. If you feel that you are at a particularly high level of risk, you should of course consider expending more time and effort to offset that risk.

Using the example of Abe and Erin from the beginning of this book, Abe invested two years of his life in the martial arts. The average life span of a male in America is 76 years (Life expectancy, 2011). In 2013, Abe was 23 years old. Those two years he invested in the martial arts bought him 53 years of expected life. In this case, Abe's investment in his survival paid enormous dividends for him as well as for the other three people he saved.

Key Points in Chapter Seven

- We are often forced to rely on prior preparation rather than logical thought processes, especially during a crisis. People in a crisis will often do exactly what they practice during a drill.
- The human mind and body react in specific, somewhat predictable ways under life and death stress.
- Training can help to overcome some of the low-level effects of crisis stress.
- Developing a plan can help you learn to react more effectively for any type of crisis. Plans needs to be technically sound and realistically practiced.
- Exposure to civil liability increases significantly in the event of serious injury or death caused by inadequate drill processes.
- It is much better to find challenges and identify solutions in advance than to work through them in the middle of a crisis.

- Take into account unique concerns and weather conditions specific to your location.
- Consider seeking assistance from someone with an emergency management background, especially if you are planning for an organization or have a family member with special needs.
- Drills and exercises should be designed to allow practice in decision making.

BIBLIOGRAPHY

Alert system fell silent during Red Lake School shooting. (2005). PostBulletin.com. Retrieved from *http://www.postbulletin.com/alert-system-fell-silent-during-red-lake-school-shooting/article_8d3095d4-38a7-58b8-84f0-4e659f963f56.html?mode=jqm*

Brendtro, L. K. (2005). The worst school violence. *Reclaiming Children and Youth, 14*(2), 73–79

Grossman, D., and L. W. Christensen. (2011). *On combat: The psychology and physiology of deadly conflict in war and peace.* Milstadt, IL: Warrior Science Publications.

Dorn, C., and S. Graves. (2010). *Lincoln County School District emergency procedures.* Atlanta, GA: Safe Havens International & The Lincoln County School District.

Dorn, M. (2012). Safe topics: The first 30 seconds. *Safe Topics.* Macon, GA: Safe Havens International.

Exercises. (2012, September 28). Retrieved July 20, 2013, from *http://www.ready.gov/business/testing/exercises*

Gladwell, Malcolm. (2005). *Blink: The power of thinking without thinking.* New York: Back Bay Books.

Kifner, J. (1998). From wild talk and friendship to five deaths in a schoolyard. *The New York Times.* Retrieved from *http://www.nytimes.com/1998/03/29/us/from-wild-talk-and-friendship-to-five-deaths-in-a-schoolyard.html?*

Klein, G. (2009). *Streetlights and shadows: Searching for the keys to adaptive decision making.* Boston Massachusetts Institute of Technology.

Life expectancy: Life expectancy by country. (2011). In G.H.O.D. Repository (Ed.), *CSV.* Geneva, Switzerland: World Health Organization.

Make a plan. (2013, June 25). Retrieved July 20, 2013, from *http://www.ready.gov/make-a-plan*

McBride, M. (2004). *The fire that will not die.* Palm Springs, CA: ETC Publications.

Ripley, A. (2008). *The unthinkable: Who survives when disaster strikes—and why.* New York: Three Rivers Press.

Sullenberger, C. (2012). *Miracle on the Hudson.* Exhibit. Carolinas Aviation Museum, Charlotte, NC.

CHAPTER EIGHT

PROGRAMMING YOUR BRAIN

Ways to prepare the most powerful survival tool known to mankind—your brain.

Had he been in many parts of Latin America, Europe, Africa, or Asia, the high school student would have been shot immediately by the police officer. During an altercation after a basketball game, the young man had fired a single shot into the pavement toward a group of three young men who were approaching him with the threat of violence. He did not want to hurt anyone, but his friend had given him the gun at the basketball game for protection, and this seemed to be just the time to use it. It even seemed to work. The three potential attackers stopped in their tracks in the parking lot outside of the Northeast High School Gymnasium.

Consumed with their mutual predicament, none of them saw the school district police officer approach. His original intent was to break up what looked like a one-sided fight, but the gunshot changed everything. From his words and his actions, it was clear that the young man did not really want to hurt anyone. Fortunately for the 15 year old, he was about to be confronted by a well-trained American law enforcement officer who was required to follow relatively restrictive rules of engagement. Using his advanced training, the officer immediately drew his pistol and used his command voice to order the suspect to drop the gun. The reaction from all four of the youths was instantaneous and obvious, each bolting in a different direction. The officer ignored the three unarmed youths and chased the suspect with the gun; radioing to dispatch "This is Unit 201. Shots fired at Northeast High School, shots fired at Northeast High School parking lot! Suspect is heading on foot toward the northwest entrance of the parking lot! Request backup!"

The officer knew that a backup cruiser would soon appear just in front of the boy and guessed at his reaction, so he came to a halt. He took aim and yelled, "STOP! Police." Everything suddenly slowed down, and his world narrowed down to the boy in his sights. His years of experience and training told him exactly what the 15-year-old boy would likely do next.

With realistic practice, our brain can actually be preprogrammed to respond to crisis events. We will share some case studies that demonstrate how simple yet practical and effective drill concepts can be used to train your brain for emergency situations. This chapter will also explain evidence and research-based concepts that have been used by U.S. Navy SEALS, SWAT teams, and other high-stress operators to prepare for battle. The chapter will include how these approaches are used in the civilian world.

How to Program Your Brain for Survival

Scenes like this one play out hundreds of times each day across the United States. Police officers in many parts of the world will still shoot anyone who dares to flee, let alone those who draw a weapon on a police officer. Law enforcement officers in the United States are held to a much higher standard when employing deadly force. For this reason, American law enforcement officers must make many challenging "shoot/don't shoot" decisions based on limited information while under intensive time pressure. Even when nonlethal weapons like pepper spray are used instead of a gun, the consequences of the use of force are enough to give most officers pause even when they are clearly justified. This makes quality training imperative so officers can react rapidly rather than hesitating to ponder the implications of the use of force. Instead, this reaction must be instantaneous.

This is one reason the officer chasing the teen gunman had trained himself to handle a gunfight through mental simulation and physical practice using hundreds, if not thousands, of gunfights. These gunfights were not against real adversaries but were simulated with interactive training that included shooting at reactive steel plates, moving targets in mock cities, video simulations, and even paintball training battles with his fellow officers. He had been through so many gunfight scenarios that his reaction was a conditioned response rather than one requiring thoughtful analysis. Under field conditions, trying to reason through the situation would not only be too slow to be effective but also more prone to error (Klein, 1998). In his department, officers practiced extensively for gunfights, since one of them had already been shot and killed in the line of duty while protecting the students of Central High School (Dorn, 2002). Since a shootout in a school is an extremely challenging proposition at best, his department spared no expense in preparing him for this moment.

The Concept of Mental Simulation

The reader may find it relevant to know that the extensive training mentioned above included practice with a variety of situations in a simulator booth with service pistol that had been equipped with a laser instead of live ammunition. In the simulator, a training officer selected a wide array of scenarios where men, women, and children would try to kill the officer with a gun, screwdriver, hammer, crow bar, or other object. He had also practiced scenarios where a suspicious person would rapidly turn and brandish a harmless object that looked similar to a weapon, or suddenly drop a gun or knife requiring the officer to hold his fire.

The computer would score each scenario with each shot fired being recorded by a laser beam emitting from the pistol. The computer could isolate each shot by individual frame and show exactly where it impacted on the person being fired at by the officer. This allows the instructor to see if an officer is shooting too fast or, more commonly, not fast enough. The computer even measured how long it took the officer to draw his or her weapon to determine if the officer might be killed or forced into a possibly avoidable gunfight by being too slow or if the officer is prone to draw his or her pistol prematurely. The computer also measured the officer's voice to determine if the officer was giving commands loud enough to be heard in a real encounter, since some officers subconsciously lower their voice during these types of situations. Indeed, one officer became so rattled that he actually dropped his gun and clutched his stomach after being shot by a virtual suspect. This type of training is used to help American police officers comply with use of force restrictions that were unimaginable in our nation in 1950 and would still be considered to be restrictive in many countries today.

The Value of Mental Simulation

Over the years, intensive legal and social transformations have taken place with major implications for anyone who wants to learn to think fast and act effectively to survive a life and death encounter. Your local police train for high stakes situations based on considerable research and evaluation of how the human brain and body works under intense stress and time pressure. The good news is that you can learn the same survival skills they and the pilot flying the plane on your next vacation both use to reduce the chances of death.

Traditionally, most firearms training for law enforcement officers focused on safety and marksmanship. Even though these topics are still covered extensively, the last four decades have seen far more focus on advanced combat tactics, decision making, and techniques for functioning under life and death stress. Combat tactics today include skills like how to draw and shoot with one arm disabled, how to draw and shoot from inside a patrol car, reloading rapidly, clearing malfunctions, and a host of other specific tactical skills.

In addition to these technical skills, decision-making training helps officers understand when they are morally and legally justified in taking a human life. If you carry, or are considering carrying, a firearm for self-defense, these same skill areas are also relevant to you, as we will describe in Chapter Nine. However, if you are like the majority of people in the United States who do not carry a firearm for protection, the other skill areas relating to decision making are still highly relevant to you. We will focus on those skills here.

Active Mental Simulation

A research-based approach, mental simulation is the process of visualizing various situations in advance. Mental simulation allows people to participate in dozens, hundreds, or even thousands of critical incidents in a relatively short period of time. For example, the school police officer faced with the "shoot/don't shoot" decision in the opening of this chapter had attended a training program at the Georgia Police Academy requiring him to run through simulated judgmental use of force scenarios for three consecutive days. His department also required him to complete a one-week refresher course on the use of force every summer. In this training, he ran through numerous scenarios using steel targets that reacted visibly and audibly when hit. Using special targets and ammunition, officers were able to duel with each other without actually shooting at one another. Each officer would shoot at rows of steel plates that, when hit, raised a target for their opponent. This activity allows officers to mentally prepare for a gunfight where they may need to react to hits by an opponent and continue firing. During this grueling week of training, officers also engaged each other in simulated gunfights using paintball rounds.

These various forms of gunfight simulation allow officers to practice the actual physical skills they would need in a gunfight, while also practicing decision making under stress. Each type of training activity is focused on instilling specific skill sets needed by officers to maximize the power of their brain in a gunfight so that decision making becomes automatic. Part of this training was designed to reinforce what the officers had been taught about continually training themselves to make life-saving decisions when an armed aggressor must be stopped. As Grossman puts it, they were trained to *live* rather than to *kill* through the use of deadly force if required (Grossman, 2008).

Passive Mental Simulation

Officers can also be trained to regularly mentally visualize different tactical situations while they are on patrol. For example, an officer driving through a downtown area at two in the morning could visualize an aggressor opening fire on him with a shotgun as he turns into an alleyway. This might require the officer to run the aggressor down with his patrol car, disengage by backing up rapidly, fire at the aggressor through the windshield, or drop down and exit the patrol car via the passenger door and return fire from behind the car door. Each of these options could be viable depending on the distance from the aggressor, layout of the alley, and a variety of other factors that would have to be evaluated in mere seconds in an actual incident. By mentally picturing themselves encountering a wide array of scenarios over time, officers build what Grossman refers to as a "mental library." According to Grossman, our brains have the ability to rapidly retrieve information that has been filed away. Grossman and other experts emphasize the need to properly prepare the brain through mental simulation (Grossman and Christensen, 2011; Klein, 2009; Ripley, 2008). Mental simulation can be performed with elaborate or relatively simple activities. A more complex form of mental simulation, and perhaps the best-known example for the average person, is the concept of flight simulator training for pilots.

Advanced Simulation Training Techniques

The pressure on a pilot and copilot when a plane full of passengers is suddenly in distress is considerable. Like law enforcement officers and soldiers, pilots simulate life and death situations using a variety of means, most notably the flight simulator. The landing of U.S. Airways flight 1549 on the Hudson River by Captain Sullenberger in 2009 is a prime example of how real-life experience combined with flight simulator training can allow people to achieve amazing successes during the most stressful of moments. This not only required a level of skill in the physical act of landing the plane on water but, just as importantly, the mental ability to stay calm in a situation where the average person might simply adopt a fatalistic numbness (Brooks et al., 2009). Any police officer or soldier who has survived a gun battle can relate that the "real deal" is different. At the same time, soldiers, law enforcement officers, and pilots who have survived these ultimate tests will typically credit their training and preparation for their ability to survive. As is often the case, these concepts have been co-opted by criminals and terrorists. The ability of the 9/11 hijackers to learn so much from flight simulator training is a stark example of the power of mental simulation.

Mental simulation takes many forms and is now used in a variety of other fields. For example, school bus drivers, teachers, school administrators, receptionists, and other school employees now use video scenario training to learn how to make life and death decisions more quickly and effectively. We train hundreds of thousands of school bus drivers, educators, school support employees, and public safety officials each year using video and scripted scenarios. More progressive school districts even run video crisis simulations in streaming format so school administrators can run different crisis simulations during each monthly staff meeting. Running scenarios on a regular basis combined with monthly Dorn Drills as described in Chapter Seven creates a desire among employees to learn the emergency protocols in their crisis plan and makes them pay attention to the locations of fire alarm pull stations, automatic external defibrillators, first-aid kits, and safe rooms where they keep their room keys and other critical items that can increase survivability when a crisis strikes without warning. This approach entails very little time relative to the substantial gains in emergency preparedness that will result.

Field-Specific Applications of Mental Simulation

As educators have adapted mental simulation to fit the school environment, appropriate approaches to mental simulation can be developed for any setting. One great thing about mental simulation is that once you have a basic scenario, you can adapt it to almost any environment. For example, one of the most challenging scenarios we have for school bus drivers is a staged scene where a student on a school bus jumps to his feet, pulls out a large semiautomatic pistol, places the muzzle of the gun to his head, and announces the he is going to kill himself. In the scene, other students on the bus appear to be in shock.

A number of students have committed suicide with guns on school property during the school day at public, parochial, and independent schools, so this is not a far-fetched scenario at all for any school anywhere in the nation. The scenario is filmed on a school bus with high school-aged student actors and a replica firearm; we have used this video to train school-based personnel as well as people who work in hundreds of different nonschool settings. By instructing participants to project the actions of the student into their own work setting and mentally changing the student into a coworker or customer, people who work in a government building, car dealership, travel agency, or any other setting can use this video to practice the skills that they would need to better address a person brandishing a gun and threatening to kill himself.

Applying Mental Simulation to Your Environment

But how can you use mental simulation if you are not an airline pilot, law enforcement officer, airborne ranger, or educator in one of these proactive schools? On an individual level, you can also use video scenarios to learn to mentally simulate an endless variety of situations. Once you have run through a series of scenarios, you can do just as law enforcement officers are trained to do and create your own scenarios in your mind. To view a series of video scenarios created to accompany this book, visit *www.SafeHavensInternational.org*.

A key point to remember is that like a law enforcement officer, you should not run scenarios with a "doomsday" mentality but rather run them in a positive way. For example, police officers are taught to visualize themselves winning a gunfight rather than being killed. Just as athletes have been trained for decades to visualize themselves getting a hole in one, a home run, or a touchdown, you should imagine yourself winning by surviving. If you find yourself worrying more after conducting mental simulations, you should carefully consider whether you have been focusing enough on running simulations with successful positive outcomes (Waitley, 1986).

When you run through the scenarios we have provided, we encourage you to see them as stepping stones to effective mental simulations rather than just a series of scenarios to watch. By creating your own scenarios, you can develop the simple habit of running through a different scenario once a week or once a month depending on what your particular risk level is. For example, if you work in a setting where you regularly interact with the public and you commonly encounter upset or angry customers, or you are in a community with a high crime rate, you might benefit from running a different simulation in your mind once a week or more. If you work somewhere with less risk, one scenario per month may be more appropriate. The key is to mentally simulate a wide array of situations on a regular and periodic basis. This allows you to develop your ability to react to danger.

Make sure that the solutions you are visualizing are appropriate and realistic. Take note of the considerations we list for each of the video scenarios, the key points of the other video segments, and of the concepts you have been learning in this book. After you have run through a simulation, mentally check your decisions against the steps in the window of life, to be fully explained later, to see if you applied each step. There are times where you should deviate from these steps to fit a particular scenario; however, this concept will apply to most situations, and you should have a good reason to deviate from them if you do so. It is also very important for you to keep a positive outlook when using mental simulations. Consciously avoid seeing the scenarios as predictive of what is likely to be. Mental simulation should reduce fear, not increase it.

Conclusion

Generally speaking, the wider the array and the greater the frequency of these exercises, the more prepared you will be for any situation you face. If there is a window of opportunity for you to survive an encounter, your chances will improve with effective and regular practice. The more emergency situations you simulate, the greater your brain's mental library to rapidly identify a viable survival strategy will be. Remember, you are programming your brain to function more effectively every time you run a mental simulation. Just as you can get better at snow skiing, boxing, tennis, or other activities requiring fast thinking and action, practice can help you get better at surviving a deadly encounter.

So how did the incident in the parking lot of Northeast High School end? It ended just as the officer thought it would. When he realized that he was trapped, the young man spun around quickly while starting to bring his gun up. A large glowing tritium blob on the front sight of the officer's duty pistol marked the youth's chest as his finger began to tighten on the trigger. Fortunately, the young man realized he would be too late to win the fight and immediately dropped the gun. The boy might have tried to shoot it out if the officer had not been demonstrably ready for the encounter when the young man made eye contact with him.

Though the officer could and would have fired if he needed to, his reaction was a conditioned response rather than a panicked one. An officer lacking the extensive training described in this chapter might have fired from fear rather than exercising the level of restraint and, more importantly, the control that years of mental simulation and live fire had created. Sometimes, the best way to win a gunfight is to prevent one in the first place. These same concepts can help you think and act faster during the window of life, too.

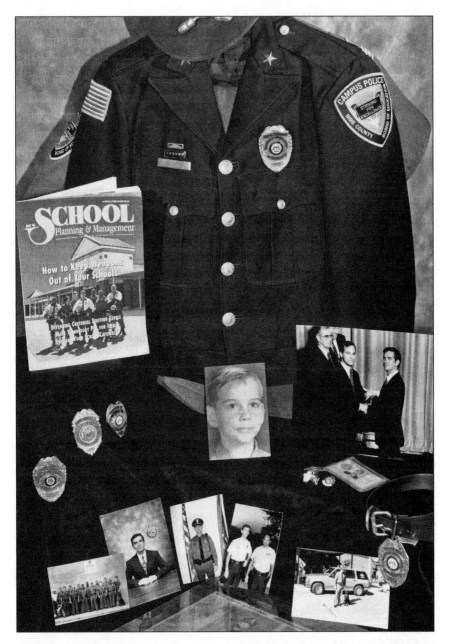

Michael Dorn, police chief: The officer in this story was coauthor Michael Dorn. Brutally raped by two boys when he was a child, then savagely bullied and attacked with a box cutter during his senior year in high school, Dorn does not allow these experiences to define who he is and does not live his life in fear. Appointed Chief of Police at the age of 27, he went on to achieve wide acclaim in his field.
Photo: Rachel Wilson

Key Points in Chapter Eight

- With realistic practice, our brain can actually be preprogrammed to respond to crisis events.
- Mental simulation is the process of visualizing various situations in advance. It allows people to react to critical incidents in a relatively short period of time to build a mental library of responses.
- Our brains have the ability to rapidly retrieve information that has been filed away. Creating a mental library to draw from in a crisis and using mental simulation can help someone respond to an emergency even if that person has never experienced one before.

BIBLIOGRAPHY

Brooks, M., J. Meserve, and M. Ahlers. (2009). Airplane crash-lands into Hudson River; all aboard reported safe. CNN.com/US. Retrieved from: *http://www. cnn.com/2009/US/01/15/new.york.plane.crash/index.html*

Dorn, M. (2012). Safe topics: The first 30 seconds. *Safe Topics*. Macon, GA: Safe Havens International.

Dorn, M. (2002). *School/law enforcement partnerships: A guide to police work in schools*. Dallas: Ram Publishing Company.

Grossman, D. (2008). The bulletproof mind: Prevailing in violent encounters . . . and after [DVD]. Delta Media.

Grossman, D., and L. W. Christensen. (2011). *On combat: The psychology and physiology of deadly conflict in war and peace*. Milstadt, IL: Warrior Science Publications.

Klein, G. (1998). *Sources of power: How people make decisions*. Cambridge, MA: The MIT Press.

Klein, G. (2009). *Streetlights and shadows: Searching for the keys to adaptive decision making*. Boston: Massachusetts Institute of Technology.

Mydans, S. (1994). Rodney King is awarded $3.8 million. *The New York Times*. Retrieved from *http://www.nytimes.com/1994/04/20/us/rodney-king-is-awarded-3.8-million.html*

Ripley, A. (2008). *The unthinkable: Who survives when disaster strikes—and why*. New York: Three Rivers Press.

Tennessee v. Garner, 471 U.S. 1(1985). Retrieved July 13, 2013, from *http:// caselaw.lp.findlaw.com/scripts/getcase.pl?navby=CASE&court=US&vol= 471&page=1*

Waitley, D. (1986). *The psychology of winning*. New York: Berkley Publishing Group.

CHAPTER NINE

IN SELF DEFENSE: IS IT LOGICAL FOR YOU TO CARRY A GUN?

Carrying a gun for protection requires thoughtful consideration and appropriate preparation.

It was mid-December, and nearly 10,000 shoppers crowded the Clackamas Town Center, a suburban mall in Portland, Oregon. Many children were excited to see Santa Claus, and the crowds were enjoying the decorations and holiday music playing over loudspeakers. Everyone seemed to be smiling, focused on their shopping.

Suddenly, a series of pops rang out. Different people identified the sounds based on their own bases of experience. A Macy's clerk thought a dress rack had fallen. Another person thought that fireworks had gone off indoors. Another in an electronics store thought it sounded like a bunch of balloons. Brance Wilson, a navy veteran and the man who was playing Santa Claus, knew they were gunshots. His base of experience told him the speed of the repeated shots indicated someone who "meant business" was firing them (Griffin, 2012).

The man who "meant business" was 22 years old. He had geared up in the mall parking lot, pulling weapons from his 1996 Volkswagen Jetta and entered Clackamas Town Center. He was wearing camouflage, a load-bearing vest some mistook for body armor, and a white hockey mask and was armed with a stolen AR-15 semiautomatic rifle with several fully loaded magazines. He walked into the mall announcing, "I am the shooter," and opened fire. He fired about 20 times before his rifle jammed (Lohr, 2012).

When the media began reporting the incident as an attack with an assault rife in a crowded mall, the world braced for yet another outcome like that of the shooting at a movie theater in Aurora, Colorado, just six months earlier. In that attack, 12 people were killed and another 70 were wounded because the killer was able to fire his weapon for an estimated seven minutes without being challenged by anyone with the capability of stopping him (Benner, 2012).

Thankfully, Nick Meli, recently credentialed as an armed security guard and concealed carry permit holder, was shopping at Clackamas Town Center with a friend and her baby when he heard the shots. The woman and her baby hit the floor as Nick took cover behind a pillar. The shooter was working on his jammed rifle as Nick drew his handgun. Seeing someone move behind his target, Nick held his fire because he knew that if he missed, he might kill an innocent person. The shooter saw him, cleared his jam, went down a utility hallway, and shot himself. Like many active shooters, the killer took his own life soon after being confronted by someone with the ability to engage him with a firearm.

Tragically, he had already killed Steven Forsyth, 45, and Cindy Yuille, 54, and seriously wounded Kristina Shevchenko, 15. This story illustrates the negative effects of a gun being used by one human being against another. This story also demonstrates how a responsible citizen with a gun can stop an armed aggressor. However, even in the hands of a responsible owner with legitimate intentions, the use of a gun can sometimes turn into a tragedy, as in the case of Jeffrey Giuliano. In the town of New Fairfield, Connecticut, Giuliano is a popular fifth-grade teacher and has a lawful permit to carry a gun. Around 1:00 A.M. on the morning of September 27, 2012, Jeffrey received a call from his sister who lived next door. Panicked, she told him that someone was attempting to break into her house. Jeffrey got his gun out and went next door to render aid. Searching the house in the dark, Jeffrey was suddenly rushed by someone wearing a mask and brandishing a knife. Reacting instinctively, Jeffrey shot the attacker in self-defense, killing him. Already distraught by the fact that he had taken someone's life, Jeffrey's anguish was intensified when it was confirmed that the "attacker" was actually his adopted son, Tyler.

We will probably never know why Tyler, whom Jeffrey had adopted four years prior, rushed out of the darkness with a knife that evening. Today, Jeffrey lives with a back injury that he suffered in the attack along with the mental trauma he experienced. When he first learned that he had killed his son, Jeffrey began weeping so uncontrollably that he began vomiting. No criminal charges were filed, and Jeffrey's back will heal, but the emotional pain will remain even though his use of a gun was justified based on the information he had at the time he fired. As with shootings by law enforcement officers, there can be tragic outcomes when a firearm is used, no matter how much care is taken to avoid it.

In these stories, we see a small part of the broad spectrum of effects of violence involving firearms. Sometimes guns are used irresponsibly to do harm. Sometimes they are used responsibly to stop harm. These incidents also usually raise questions about whether civilians should have guns or not. Although the topic is a highly controversial, politically loaded, and often very emotional issue, the fact remains that approximately 112 million people in the United States own a firearm, and more than 75 million Americans report owning a firearm for self-defense (Carroll, 2005).

This chapter was written because no matter how you feel about the gun control debate, millions of Americans do own a firearm for protection. While the discussion on gun control is a healthy and necessary part of democracy, the fact remains that approximately one in three American adults owns a gun for protection (General demographic, 2005). In this chapter, we will attempt to provide readers with logical and measured guidance on when and where carrying a gun can reduce their risk of death as well as when this approach might be inappropriate. We will also try to help readers understand the limitations that firearms have as self-defense tools. There are also a number of critical technical points that should be carefully considered and addressed before a civilian carries a firearm. Martial arts and personal safety devices, like Mace, pepper spray, impact weapons, stun guns, Tasers, and other self-protection devices will also be explored.

Is It Logical for You?

After experiencing the terrifying hatchet attack we described at the beginning of this book, Abe and Erin began to seriously consider their defense options. What they did not do is immediately go out and buy a gun. The first question anyone should ask when making a decision to obtain a gun for self-defense is whether or not he or she feels confident to take a human life if necessary. This is one of the most serious actions a human being can take. If this is not something that you feel comfortable doing, no other considerations matter. This decision should be made before, not during, a violent incident. Hesitation during an attack could mean missing the chance to take action, or more importantly it could give your attacker the chance to use your own weapon against you.

The use of a gun comes with permanent consequences that involve the immersion into what Lt. Col. Grossman calls the "Universal Phobia." Grossman emphasizes that committing the ultimate violence—taking a life—carries with it long-term emotional, and possibly physical, consequences for the person who uses the gun as well as the person who gets shot. Using a gun to protect yourself is very different than in the movies. Many police officers and soldiers have learned the hard way that they were not prepared to kill. When coauthor Michael Dorn attended an 11-week training program at the FBI National Academy at Quantico, Virginia, he was surprised to learn how many FBI Agent recruits quit the academy because they realized that they might actually be required to take a human life.

The second question to ask of yourself is whether you are likely to need a gun or not. This is a complex question with numerous variables to consider. The biggest factor to consider is your actual level of danger. Living or working in a high crime area can increase the practicality of carrying a firearm. Specific interpersonal situations can also impact this type of decision. If you have cause to be concerned about someone who might try to attack or kill you, carrying a firearm may be a logical choice. While many experts maintain that you are more likely to be disarmed by an aggressor than to successfully protect yourself, thousands of people have successfully used guns to protect themselves without this happening.

When researching these statistics, it is important not to rely only on data that only counts fatalities and to consider the context of each study. There are now multiple peer-reviewed studies that demonstrate that in most instances where a gun is used for self-defense, no one gets shot. Twice each year, the U.S. Bureau of Justice Statistics conducts a national survey of household crime to create a crime index. One analysis of these data showed that among incidents of gun use in self-defense, less than 1 percent of cases resulted in the gun being taken away from the owner. This same analysis revealed that the rate of injury dropped from 25 percent to 17 percent in cases where a gun was used in defense (Kleck, 1997). Coauthor Michael Dorn has experienced this multiple times in situations where an aggressor backed down as soon as the aggressor became aware that he was carrying or had drawn a gun.

Another reason to carry a gun might be when you have a job that creates the need for this type of protection. For example, some real estate professionals work in high-crime neighborhoods each day while other people have jobs that require them to transport large amounts of cash. These people may opt to carry a gun for self-defense. Many off-duty police officers carry a gun even when these types of risks are not present because they are specially trained and prepared to protect others.

Important Considerations for Carrying a Gun

Carrying a gun involves a number of responsibilities. One does not simply walk into a store and buy a gun and become instantly protected. In order to properly and safely carry a gun, you need to consider other factors thoughtfully, including legality, liability, the type of gun and ammunition, and safe storage and carry as well as training and practice. Detailed discussion of these topics is beyond the scope of this book; however, there are a number of important questions you should ask yourself before buying any type of self-defense equipment:

- What type of weapon is practical and safe for you to carry?
- What type of ammunition will provide adequate protection while not creating increased risks for others?
- How will you safely store and transport the weapon?
- How will you carry the weapon effectively and safely?
- What kind of training should you have and how often should you train?
- What are the legal concerns related to carrying the weapon?
- What type of liability insurance coverage should you have in relation to the use of a weapon?
- Are you prepared for the legal and moral implications of using the weapon?

If you decide that it is appropriate for you to carry a gun, consider each of these questions and do the appropriate research. As with any security technology, the biggest factor in the success of the equipment is the level of preparation, training, and confidence of the user. As countless news stories and the killing of Trayvon Martin and the subsequent trial of George Zimmerman demonstrated, carrying a firearm can have complex repercussions.

One of the most important considerations from the questions above is the safe storage of any weapons that are not actively in use. Owning a gun entails a significant responsibility for safety. This means not only safe handling of the weapon and ammunition but storage as well. There have even been cases where children have accidentally set off ammunition by tapping on the primer. These risks are even higher if there are children in the area where the weapon will be carried or stored, or if the area is frequented by adults who are irresponsible due to mental capacity or character. An example would be if you were caring for a family member who has Alzheimer's or has a history of being careless. Though accidental deaths involving firearms have declined and are relatively rare, even well-behaved children can allow curiosity to overcome parental warnings relating to firearms safety. As with the other considerations we have discussed, be sure to conduct research and make a well-informed decision.

As a final caution, having a gun can sometimes subconsciously influence people to put themselves in dangerous situations because of the feeling of security that a firearm can provide. For example, do not walk down a dark alley in a high-crime area that you would normally avoid if you were not carrying a gun. Avoid altercations and dangerous individuals just like you would as if you were unarmed. A gun is a useful tool to help you survive bad situations, but it does not guarantee that you will not be attacked. Remember that you will survive 100 percent of the situations you do not get into (Givens, 2013).

For more discussion on the questions above and for suggestions on how to answer them, view the supplemental article for this chapter, "Important Considerations Before Carrying a Gun" at *www.SafeHavensInternational.org.*

Alternatives to Carrying a Gun

Carrying a gun is not an appropriate option for everyone. If you decide that it would not be a good choice for you, there are alternative defensive force options. We suggest you still consider these even if you do carry a firearm. Indeed, choosing to carry a gun does not mean that a person cannot learn martial arts or how to use alternative defensive weapons. Sometimes people are assaulted in a manner that does not lawfully or morally justify the use of deadly force.

Unarmed Combat

Like carrying a firearm, martial arts are not appropriate for many people. It is important to understand that martial arts techniques have significant limitations in many situations, especially those where an aggressor is armed with a gun or a knife. There is no reliable technique for an unarmed person to disarm someone with a knife or gun without putting him- or herself at extreme risk.

In fact, trying to defend yourself without the proper training can increase your risk of injury or death. In a study of gas station robberies in Florida in the 1990s, it was found that the risk of injury increased by more than 80 percent when resistance was offered during a robbery. Analysis of other studies from this same data set indicate that no matter how many clerks were working at the time of the robbery or what security technologies or practices were in place, the training of the clerks is one of the most likely ways to reduce the chances of injury (Atlas, 2013).

In the hatchet attack, Abe's martial arts skills allowed him to defeat an attacker who was armed and violent. Abe felt he had forgotten everything he had learned, but in fact he did benefit from the muscle memory and physical concentration that his two years of *Songham Taekwondo* provided. He was able to disarm his attacker twice and then deliver a decisive blow to his attacker's groin that conclusively stopped the attack and caused the aggressor to flee the scene. This is a perfect example of how the specific techniques Abe used were less important than the overall level of ability to use his body as a defensive weapon.

There are a number of martial arts forms originating in different cultures from around the world, each with its own strengths and weaknesses. As with the selection of a firearm, we suggest you carefully research whether martial arts training is a practical choice for you. If you decide to learn any of the martial arts, you should also carefully research where you will take martial arts training. Martial arts training also requires a significant time commitment. However, as many martial artists will relate, there are numerous benefits to the training. Many people find martial arts to be an enjoyable way to build self-discipline and practice physical and mental conditioning.

"Close-in" Weapons

Many of the formal martial arts include some forms of weapons training. These weapons are often either edged weapons like knives, swords, and spears or impact weapons like the staff (*bō*), a pair of nun-chucks (*nunchaku*), or blunt-force weapons. The purpose of this is to teach discipline while handling any type of weapon, and to strengthen the mind and body through repetition—the same repetition that saved Abe's life.

Sticks have been used as tools and weapons in some form or fashion since the dawn of man. The use of these types of weapons can seem almost instinctive. For example, many people keep a baseball bat near the front door to use as a weapon against a violent intruder. It is important to keep in mind that the legal guidelines for the use of deadly force are the same whether you use a gun, a bat, or a kitchen knife. It is also important to understand the limitations of any type of weapon. Just as a person should not carry a firearm unless he is mentally prepared to use it to take a human life, it can be a very bad idea to plan to use any other type of weapon that can be used against you if you are not ready, willing, and able to use it defensively.

Knives are also considered "close-in" weapons because to use them you have to violently invade someone's personal space. Knives can also do quite a bit of damage in a short amount of time, and many people are killed with knives every year. According to the FBI, 1,659 people were murdered with knives and other edged weapons in the United States in 2011 (FBI, 2012). More people are killed with simple pocketknives each year than most people realize. As we have pointed out in other chapters, approximately 200 people have been killed and injured in mass casualty stabbing incidents in K–12 schools in China in recent years. As but one example, in April 2013, one student killed another student with a pocketknife at Cleveland High School in Reseda, California (Serna, 2013).

Many people carry knives for self-defense and utility. Once we train people in visual weapons screening techniques, they are often astounded at how many people they spot who are carrying some form of edged weapon. Modern knife catalogues contain hundreds of options. There are myriad training programs and videos available on the use of knives for self-defense. So is a knife a viable option for self-defense?

We are hesitant to recommend a knife as a self-defense weapon. The most compelling limitation of a knife as a self-defense weapon for the average person is that knives typically do not deter or neutralize an armed attacker as effectively as a firearm. While brandishing a gun might deter most attackers, many aggressors will be more likely to press an attack when threatened with a knife, and even though a well-trained and practiced person with an edged weapon can be deadly, the way knives work in life and death situations is simply not on par with firearms.

As with a gun, there are numerous legal restrictions on carrying and using an edged weapon for self-defense. Most states prohibit the concealed carry of a variety of edged weapons, and concealed weapons permits typically only authorize you to carry a firearm.

New Weapons Technologies

Technological advances have given us more choices in the use of less-than-lethal weapons. From the development of things like pepper spray to the onset of "stun" weapons, we have developed better ways to protect ourselves than ever before. As with all weapons, understanding the weapon and being trained in its use will help develop responsible use. These options also have their limitations and legal restrictions. It is also important to remember that just because a weapon is considered "nonlethal" does not mean that serious injury or death cannot result from its use.

Pepper Spray

Pepper spray is one of the most popular forms of nonlethal self-defense items. Mace is a common name for this broad spectrum of chemical sprays used for self-defense. It was first created in 1965 from an aerosolized mixture of phenacyl chloride, also known as CN (Blain, 2003). Because of the potential toxic nature of CN, most mixtures now use an oleoresin capsicum (OC) mixture (Vesaluoma, et al., 2000). Pepper spray often has a powerful effect on people who are sprayed with it.

Pepper spray is also marketed as "bear spray" for hikers and campers to carry in case of a bear attack. Jack Hanna, the famous animal expert, successfully used pepper spray against a grizzly bear in Glacier National Park in Montana. He and his wife were hiking a well-known trail when they met a group of fellow hikers. Just then a mother grizzly with a yearling approached, putting all of the hikers in serious danger. Grizzlies run too fast for humans to outrun them, so Hanna used bear spray. His first spray was blown away by the wind, so he had to wait until the mother grizzly was incredibly close to him to engage her with the rest of the canister. This caused the mother enough discomfort that she ran away, saving Jack, his wife, and the other hikers (Olivares, 2010).

Like other types of weapons, there are numerous instances where bears and people who have been sprayed with pepper spray are able to continue their aggression. In a controlled experiment, Sergeant Steve Meadows with the Bibb County Public School System Police Department was able to draw his pistol from a holster and fire 52 rounds into the kill zone of a police-training target after being heavily sprayed with police issue pepper spray. This required him to change magazines twice and then resume firing each time.

As a police officer, coauthor Michael Dorn has personally seen pepper spray fail to incapacitate aggressors on more than one occasion. We should point out to the reader that there are also examples of people who have been shot with firearms and not immediately incapacitated. There is also a risk of the spray being blown toward you, causing symptoms in yourself instead of your intended target. We do not mean to imply that pepper spray is not effective, but rather we want to familiarize the reader with its limitations, particularly in instances where an aggressor is armed. We do not feel that pepper spray is a reliable means to counter an attacker with a firearm, edged weapon, or impact weapon. At the same time, it can be used to effectively deter an unarmed aggressor if properly applied with the right coordinated action on the part of the victim.

"Stun Guns" and Tasers

There have also been advancements in weapons that operate with electrical shocks. These include stun guns (devices that require direct physical contact with the target to work) and Tasers, which fire a set of prongs with thin wires connecting them to the device. Stun guns are pain producing, used as a means of forcing compliance, while Tasers deliver a powerful shock through the prongs that create neuromuscular interference, incapacitating the target while the current is flowing.

Stun guns have the distinct limitation of requiring a user to be able to physically touch the aggressor with the weapon. While this may work for an unarmed attacker, this type of device is of limited use against anyone who is armed, especially if the aggressor has a firearm. Even though Tasers also have limitations, many law enforcement officers carry them so that they have a less lethal option for neutralizing aggressive suspects. As law enforcement officers are trained not to rely on Tasers to counter an assault with a firearm, we too are reluctant to suggest the Taser as suitable for personal defense against someone who is armed with a firearm, knife, or other deadly weapon.

Any weapon you choose, be it firearms, martial arts, or nonlethal weapons will require careful deliberation, extensive training, and mental preparation. People who are not mentally and physically prepared can create a bigger risk for themselves and others if they carry a weapon that can be used against them. There is also a risk of escalating the situation if an attacker feels threatened. For example, in some cases, victims who threaten an attacker with nonlethal weapons have prompted the attacker to pull a gun or knife in response.

Conclusion

There are a number of options for defending yourself. Although there is currently no more reliable way than a firearm to stop a determined and armed aggressor, this choice is not practical, legal, or appropriate for everyone. For those who are considering whether carrying a gun is appropriate or not, we urge a pragmatic and thorough consideration of the matter, starting with what can quickly become the most important question: whether or not you are confident that you could take a human life. For those who have already made this decision after weighing the considerations, we urge lawful, thoughtful, and responsible gun ownership. This requires adequate safety training; attention to legal considerations; adequate practice; careful selection of firearms, ammunition, and holsters; and a safe approach to storage of firearms and ammunition.

Coauthor Michael Dorn has survived a number of attacks with guns, box cutters, knives, and even a bayonet. In one incident, two men who were walking toward him crossed the street to approach him while he was jogging at night. In response, Dorn crossed to the other side of the street. When he did so, both men crossed the street as well and appeared to be looking around for potential witnesses. When Dorn crossed the street a third time, the two men did likewise and were only about 30 yards in front of him. Now convinced that he was about to be attacked, Dorn drew his handgun and the men quickly crossed to the other side of the street again and continued on their way. Two men closely fitting their description robbed another pedestrian about 15 minutes later a few blocks from where this confrontation occurred.

These and other experiences taught him that firearms, pepper spray, impact devices, and other protective tools can prevent death. They have also taught him that the other survival concepts described throughout this book are always at least as important as any weapon one might carry.

Key Points in Chapter Nine

- A responsible citizen with a gun can often stop an armed aggressor without firing a single shot, but in some cases carrying a gun may not be your best option.
- Hesitation during an attack could mean missing the chance to take action or give your attacker the chance to use your own weapon against you. If you carry a gun, be prepared to act, and act fast.
- Owning a gun entails a significant responsibility for the safety of those around you, including from harm by attackers as well as accidents.
- Firearms training should also be approached in a thoughtful, thorough manner. Be prepared to take the time to practice extensively and periodically if you carry any kind of weapon.
- Having a gun or other weapon should not mean that you put yourself in dangerous situations.
- A gun is a useful tool to help you survive bad situations, but it does not guarantee that you will not be attacked.
- There is no reliable technique for an unarmed person to disarm someone with a knife or gun without putting him- or herself at extreme risk.
- It can be a very bad idea to plan to use any type of weapon that can be used against you if you are not ready, willing, and able to use it defensively.

BIBLIOGRAPHY

Atlas, R. I. (2013). *21st Century Security and CPTED: Designing for Critical Infrastructure Protection and Crime Prevention* (2nd ed.). Boca Raton, FL: CRC Press.

Benner, J. (2012). Colorado tragedy: Dark knight rises massacre. Retrieved from *http://joshbenner.org/2012/07/20/colorado-tragedy-dark-knight-rises-massacre/*

Blain, P. G. (2003). Tear gases and irritant incapacitants: 1-chloroacetophenone, 2-chlorobenzylidene malononitrile and dibenz [B,F]-1,4-oxazepine. *Toxicological Reviews, 22*(2), 103–110.

Carroll, J. (2005). Gun ownership and use in America. Gallup Poll. Retrieved from *http://www.gallup.com/poll/20098/gun-ownership-use-america.aspx*

Expanded homicide data table 8. (2009). Murder victims by weapon (Ed.). Washington, DC: U.S. Department of Justice.

FBI: Law enforcement officers feloniously killed and assaulted: Percent distribution by time of incident, 2002–2011. (2012). In F. 1 (Ed.), *Excel*. Washington, DC: Federal Bureau of Investigation.

General demographic characteristics (2005). Washington, DC: U.S. Census Bureau.

Givens, T. (2013, February). Become an "A" student. *Concealed Carry Magazine, 10*.

Griffin, A. (2012). *Clackamas Town Center shooting: 22 minutes of chaos and terror as a gunman meanders through the mall*. The Oregonian. December 16, 2012. Retrieved from *http://www.oregonlive.com/clackamascounty/index.ssf/2012/12/clackamas_town_center_shooting_61.html*

Gun ownership statistics and demographics. (2013). Retrieved June 26, 2013, from *http://www.statisticbrain.com/gun-ownership-statistics-demographics/*

James, F. (2004). *Effective handgun defense: A comprehensive guide to concealed carry*. Iola, WI: Krause Publications.

Kleck, G. (1997). *Guns and self defense*. Retrieved from *http://www.pulpless.com/gunclock/kleck2.html*

Law enforcement officers feloniously killed with own weapons: Victim officer's type of weapon 2002–2011. (2012). In T. 14 (Ed.), *Excel*. Washington, DC: Federal Bureau of Investigation.

Lohr, D. (2012). *Jacob Tyler Roberts identified as Clackamas town center shooter*. The Huffington Post. Retrieved from *http://www.huffingtonpost.com/2012/12/12/clackamas-town-center-shooting_n_2283795.html*

Olivares, X. (2010). Zookeeper Jack Hanna uses pepper spray to save hikers from a bear. ABC News. Retrieved from *http://abcnews.go.com/WN/zookeeper-jack-hanna-pepper-spray-save-hikers-bear/story?id=11263009#.UdOjkOuvt7Y*

Serna, J. (2013). 2 arrested in stabbing death of Cleveland High student in Reseda. *LA Times*. Retrieved April 25, 2013, from *http://articles.latimes.com/2013/apr/25/local/la-me-ln-cleveland-high-school-stabbing-20130425*

Street smarts: How Mace protected Heather. (2013). Retrieved July 2, 2013, from *http://www.mace.com/story-heatherhttp://www.mace.com/story-heather*

Upson, S. (2007). How a taser works. *IEEE Spectrum*. Retrieved from *http://spectrum.ieee.org/consumer-electronics/gadgets/how-a-taser-works*

Vesaluoma, M., J. Gallar, A. Lambiase, J. Moilanen, T. Hack, C. Belmonte, and T. Tervo. (2000). Effects of oleoresin capsicum pepper spray on human corneal morphology and sensitivity. *Investigative Ophthalmology & Visual Science, 41*(8), 2138–2147.

CHAPTER TEN

THE FIRST 30 SECONDS— THE CRITICAL WINDOW OF LIFE

Or how to make faster and more effective decisions in the first critical seconds of a life-threatening event.

On November 4, 1994, a deafening explosion rocked Charlton County High School in rural south Georgia. Twelve students were injured, with three of them in critical condition. The investigation by the Georgia Bureau of Investigation revealed that a student had dropped what he thought was a harmless dummy military training round on the floor of his classroom. In reality, it was a powerful and deadly piece of unexploded military ordinance designed specifically to kill and maim grown men. Military personnel brought in to help identify the device told school officials that the detonation of such a round in this type of confined space typically increases the lethality of the round. Remarkably, not one child died in this horrific accident. The decisions and communications made by school staff in the first critical moments of this crisis are an amazing testament to the ability of well-prepared people to save lives.

In an interview several months after the incident, public safety officials told one of the coauthors that the preincident planning and prompt actions of school officials once the crisis began were the deciding factors. The responding agencies had no doubt that several of the students in that classroom would have surely been killed if school officials had not done such extensive planning. This included developing specific plans and even plotting coordinates for a helipad for Medevac helicopters in case of a mass casualty event at the school.

These planning activities were not done on a whim or by luck. The school principal knew that there was limited local capacity for critical care patients, and emergency medical services were limited in the rural community. Just as importantly, when the principal reacted to what he thought was a shooting, a staff member immediately communicated that something had exploded. The principal trusted the staff member and quickly made a decision to evacuate the entire school.

When we contrast this terrifying incident and the Our Lady of Angels (OLA) school fire in 1958, the difference in outcomes is stark. Both incidents must have been truly frightening and shocking for those involved, but the fire was much deadlier than the explosion because of a fundamental difference in the decisions made by school staff during the Window of Life. An underlying cause for the reactions of staff members was the level of employee empowerment when it came to life and death situations.

Even though all of the employees at OLA practiced evacuations often and with a focus on the specific type of event they eventually experienced, staff were not properly empowered to take simple and obvious independent actions. As a result, 95 people died in an event they had all practiced for repeatedly and frequently. Conversely, the school staff at Charlton County High School made sound decisions in the first critical minutes of the incident and saved every life at risk in spite of the fact that the incident was something they had not specifically practiced for—even once. These two incidents illustrate how crucial it is to make appropriate decisions within the first 30 seconds of an emergency situation. While the actual window of time will vary depending on the incident, the chances of survival are often determined by the actions and decisions made within roughly the first 30 seconds or so of the detection of danger. This chapter discusses the techniques that can help you make the necessary critical decisions to save lives and reduce injury.

The Critical Impact of Speed

When it comes to making effective crisis decisions, speed is a critical factor. Obviously it is important to respond to an emergency quickly, most people cannot comprehend the speed of a crisis until they experience one themselves. In addition to the need to make decisions quickly, the quality of the decisions made is equally critical. As in the OLA fire, some staff members had *made decisions,* but they were not the best options to reduce the loss of life.

We developed a concept called the *Window of Life* to help explain a simple process for acting effectively when there is limited time to think, act, and communicate. The four steps in the Window of Life are:

1. protect yourself,
2. protect others in your immediate area,
3. protect the place, and then
4. notify public safety, calling 911 or other emergency services as appropriate.

These are the basic critical actions that need to be performed in a very short window of time—in the first moments of an incident—in order to save lives.

Even the most effective actions may be useless if they are just a few seconds too late. When this period has passed, the opportunity to take protective actions can be forever lost. One of the starkest examples is a lockdown during a school shooting. If the instruction to lockdown is made quickly enough, an active shooter in a school building might be presented with few if any victims to target. If there is a delay of 10 to 30 seconds in lockdown implementation, administrators may be unable to access the intercom to call a lockdown, leaving staff members exposed and potentially without any warning to the school.

In an emergency, quickly deciding which actions to take first can improve your chances of survival. Take personal protective action first, then warn others around you when it is safe to do so. If possible, warn and protect others in and around the building or space and then call 911 or emergency services as soon as you can. If you have the help of others, delegate action to get help more quickly. Use your judgment to determine the priority of your actions, since each situation will require a unique response.

www.SafeHavensInternational.org

This window of life can be a mere two seconds, or it can be longer. If you are in a public place and a person opens fire in close proximity to you, you may only have a few seconds to take action to protect yourself. If you are in that same public place and a man starts choking on food, you may have 30 to 45 seconds to make your decision to instruct someone to call 911 and attempt the Heimlich maneuver. In addition, the time frame will feel more compressed in the first instance because you have to act fast to save yourself while you are in no personal danger in the second scenario.

In some cases, this window of time will seem so narrow as to feel nonexistent. For example, if you are driving on the interstate and a large vehicle traveling 100 feet in front of you overturns, you may have a split second to take as much protective action as possible. This is also an example of a situation that could have potentially been prevented through mitigation measures, in this case, staying far behind other vehicles. Of course this is not always possible, so it is even more critical to be prepared to react instantaneously to these types of events.

Returning to the lockdown example, we have found incredible delays in the decision to call a lockdown during multiple school shooting cases that we have worked. In many cases, after-incident investigations have found that a lockdown is not ordered for anywhere from one minute to as long as eight minutes after initial shots have been fired. This can occur for a variety of reasons. In some instances, school officials heard gunshots in their school but did not recognize the sound as gunfire. In other cases, school officials became predisposed to expect certain things if a school shooting occurred, adapting a sort of fatalistic mindset.

For example, many people assume that in a school shooting there will be multiple victims, that they will hear many gunshots, and that there will be copious amounts of blood. This problem became evident during the forensic evaluation of the case of a shooting at a high school in Florida. In this incident, school staff were apparently so conditioned to think of school shootings in terms of "active shooters" that they did not realize a student had even been shot. Since no staff members were supervising the area where the student was shot, no employees heard the single gunshot from a small handgun. A responding administrator mistakenly assumed the victim had simply passed out and did not recognize that the girl had been shot, since there was very little bleeding.

Because the administrator misread the situation and thought the girl had simply passed out, there was an estimated eight-minute delay before she called for an ambulance. The 911 dispatch was first notified that there had been a shooting when they received a call from the shooter, who wanted to make sure an ambulance was on the way. The shooter was a female student with mental illness who shot a friend of hers without intending to kill her. The school system's insurance carrier opted to settle the civil case before a trial was even scheduled. These common examples of plan failure can occur in other settings like malls, churches, office buildings, and factories.

As we will discuss later in this chapter, a lack of empowerment can quickly result in lengthy and deadly delays. Perhaps one of the most common reasons for these delays in shooting incidents is the reliance upon drills that do not require any decision making by line-level staff. Conducting regular lockdown drills helps staff practice the physical action steps for a lockdown, but these traditional drills do little to mentally prepare employees to make the lockdown decision quickly without direction. Using the concept of the OODA loop, traditional drills do not simulate a realistic OODA loop for staff members, meaning staff are less likely to recognize danger and take action if they do not participate in these types of drills.

In other cases, the announcement to lock down has been delayed because office staff attempted to call 911 to report the emergency before taking any other action, not realizing that this can result in a one- to two-minute delay. This, in turn, can expose everyone in the building to danger long enough for mass casualties to occur. We must remember that even if an armed officer is on campus, it can sometimes take one or more minutes for an officer to reach the location of the incident, even while running across a small campus. This means that many victims can be injured, and even killed, whereas they might otherwise be protected if a lockdown announcement is made before the call to 911.

A lockdown announcement can be made in a few seconds, so the 911 call will likely only be minimally delayed in this course of action. If multiple staff are on duty in the office and they are prepared to work as a team without specific direction, the lockdown announcement and the call to 911 can be made simultaneously. In schools that do not have this level of preparation, staff assume that this type of reaction will occur naturally, but in a real crisis they find that not having clearly defined roles and systems can quickly result in panic.

Another element that can affect the speed of decision making during a crisis is a lack of information. Most of the decisions made in these first 30 seconds are made with limited information. In Charlton County, school staff had limited information when they told the administrator that there had been an explosion rather than a shooting. In this particular case, the nature of the incident was even more prone to cause a feeling of sensory overload and confusion because an explosion in a school would take anyone by surprise. In general, it is absolutely critical to make decisions within the first few moments of the first signs of danger. The longer the delay in making the necessary decisions, the less chance you have to save lives or reduce the negative impact of an incident.

Order of Actions

A typical response to an emergency situation involves multiple courses of action. But how can you determine which steps should be taken first and which should be implemented last? The Window of Life, as described above, not only emphasizes how short a time span we may have to take action but also shows what a typical ordering of actions in the first critical seconds of an incident looks like. We focus on the ordering of the first few action steps because this is especially critical during mass casualty events like a fire, tornado, or an active shooter.

The concept also emphasizes that you need to protect yourself first so you can more effectively protect others. This is simply an extension of how public safety officials are trained. Emergency responders are all taught in basic training that their first responsibility in a life and death situation is to protect themselves so they will then be in a position to protect other people. This message is typically reiterated as public safety officials undergo advanced training over the course of their careers. This message is normally repeated not only during training but also in the simulations of tactical situations that are a typical part of this type of training. Police officers in particular are well aware that by failing to protect themselves, officers can in turn fail in their responsibility to protect their colleagues and citizens.

The concept is very similar to what we are told to do in the event of the loss of cabin pressure in a commercial airline. Passengers are instructed to put their own mask on first before they assist others because passengers may lose consciousness and in turn not be able to help their child. However, it is very easy to forget this when the safety of those we love is involved. This is especially true when young children are at risk, even when they are not our own.

If you ask well-trained police officers what their first responsibility is during a life and death situation, they will typically tell you that it is to protect themselves so they can in turn protect others. However, when you ask educators what their first responsibility is in a life and death situation, they will invariably tell you that it is to protect their students, even if it means putting their own safety at risk. Without specific training to the contrary, this is a natural and understandable assumption for any educator. This has been greatly exacerbated by the manner in which the media covered the tragedy at Sandy Hook Elementary School in Newtown, Connecticut.

One of the predominant themes of the media coverage of that event was the bravery of school employees who placed their lives at risk to try to protect the children. Although we all can obviously respect the valor of these dedicated and caring people, we must be cautious about the resulting messages we convey to school employees. Just as police officers are carefully trained that the decision to place themselves in harm's way is a logical response based on their extensive training for these types of situations, educators should be trained to override their natural emotional response to put themselves in danger to protect others. As with public safety officials, educators who place themselves in harm's way can at times expose the children they care so deeply about to injury or death.

The barrage of media coverage focusing on the bravery of school employees at Sandy Hook has had a negative effect on the decision-making ability of many school officials around the country. Within weeks, our analysts began to notice a dramatic change in the way educators responded to our scenarios. The number of ineffective responses we have observed since the shooting in Newtown has been nothing less than disturbing. For example, we have noted that a startling number of school employees have failed to take simple and effective measures to protect students because they immediately decide that they should attack an aggressor or try to use themselves as a diversion to allow students to reach safety on their own. This type of approach would actually be less effective at protecting students in most situations. A number of the educators that we interact with have made comments to us that the Sandy Hook incident had taught them that it was now their job to die to protect students. One of the coauthors worked with a school district that was trying to decide how best to implement facilities changes and building renovations to improve safety in the district. One of the principals interviewed as part of this project ignored the initial questions we posed about the building design to state that his main concern was "Knowing what to do in the precious first few seconds of an active shooter event, since I'm going to die, and my front office staff are going to die, too." There was no doubt in this administrator's mind that sacrificing himself was a necessity if extreme violence took place on campus. Police chiefs across the country would be deeply troubled by similar state-ments if they were made by police officers in their department. Any school superintendent or headmaster should be just as concerned if district administrators go to work each day with this mindset.

These controlled simulations have demonstrated that school employees who are focused on preparing to thrust themselves into danger in a noble effort to protect others often fail to think in terms of basic and effective protective actions like implementing a lockdown. For example, using the Window of Life concept, a school office staff member who is posed with a scenario of an armed aggressor in the main office can quickly direct others to clear the room, retreat to a properly prepared safe room, lock the door, order a lockdown to protect the rest of the school, and call 911 from a position of relative safety.

We have found that school officials who are prepared to sacrifice themselves to protect students often forget that the most effective way of protecting the students under their care is to retreat to a safe area where the crisis can be handled while in lockdown. Interviews with these staff typically reveal that their first, and in many cases only, response is to place themselves in harm's way. One other exam-ple from our scenario simulations is an aggressive dog that enters the campus and approaches students. Many staff members we interview state that they would send the students inside while placing them-selves in danger by approaching the dog and in some cases attempt-ing to fight the dog. When educators focus their efforts and energy on confronting the aggressive dog, they are not able to effectively facilitate the process of getting students to safety and notifying the office so that other school staff can avoid the dangerous situation. In many cases, confronting the dog might exacerbate the situation if the dog has not yet started attacking anyone.

Keep in mind that even though the media may focus intensively on mass casualty shootings, the attack on Abe in Chapter One is a far more typical weapons assault, even though the attacker used a rather unique combination of weapons. As we have pointed out, more people are killed with hammers than with rifles in the United States. When we consider that the vast majority of attacks with firearms involves single-victim attacks, it is even more important to keep in mind that you should be prepared to protect yourself and others from the most common forms of lethal violence rather than only those that make the news. Even though mass casualty shootings are more frightening and thus popular with media outlets, they are statistically quite rare given the immense population of the United States. If you fall in the ocean in most parts of the world, there is a small chance that a shark could attack you, but the risk that you will drown if you do not know how to swim and are not wearing a life preserver is usually much higher. Spending a lot of time learning what to do if a shark attacks you while ignoring the importance of learning how to swim before embarking on a sailing trip would not be very logical either.

Another benefit of the Window of Life is that it can be applied to any life and death situation. For example, if you are outside of your place of work and spot a tornado approaching the building at a distance, utilizing the Window of Life will help protect you, others in the building, and the community at large. One of our crisis scenarios presents educators with a tornado approaching their school from a distance of 1,000 yards while they are outside supervising children. Most educators we interviewed do think to move students indoors quickly and direct them to shelter in the closest appropriate shelter area. At the same time, a startling number forget to notify anyone else in the building that a tornado is approaching.

In this example, the small percentage of school employees who think to communicate the danger most often say they would call 911. This means that the principal might not learn that there is a tornado until it hits the school. If staff members are trained to protect themselves first, protect those in the immediate area next, protect the place, and then call 911 once the other steps are initiated, they can move themselves and the students to shelter, call the office so the rest of the people in the school can take shelter, and then notify 911. As the school office should also be calling 911, this approach will provide redundant communications to increase the chances that the 911 center will receive all critical information. Many people incorrectly assume that they will not experience a tornado before public safety officials provide a warning. While warning systems have become fairly sophisticated and reliable in many parts of the country, it is still very possible for a tornado to form and do severe damage before a warning can be issued.

Perhaps the biggest challenge for people who are considering how to apply the Window of Life involves calling 911. We have become so conditioned to call 911 as soon as we detect an emergency that it is very easy to forget that there may be other protective actions that must be taken first in some situations. A police officer who is being shot at by a suspect three feet away will pull and use his service pistol before calling for assistance on the radio. As with police officers, your odds of survival will go up if you take immediate action to prevent imminent harm before calling 911—unless you can do both at the same time.

Give Yourself Permission to Live: The Benefits of Individual Empowerment

Successful crisis response at the organizational level requires people to be empowered not only to make decisions to save human lives but also to deviate from established plans and procedures to do so. This was a deadly factor in the OLA school arson attack and, as we shall see later, was apparently a critical factor in a tragic mass casualty shooting at the Red Lake Reservation in Minnesota. Under the extremely powerful effects of stress we have discussed, we can see how soldiers and law enforcement officers, let alone people who do not typically have to address life and death situations, can get locked into following plans or procedures that are not appropriate for a specific situation. Empowering staff to take independent action to prevent these types of stress reactions is what we refer to as "Permission to Live."

Simply put, Permission to Live is a mindset where people are not only empowered but also expected to take immediate action to save lives. The concept predisposes people to take immediate life-saving action without being told to do so. For this to work, people must clearly understand that they should deviate from established norms, policies, procedures, or practices *if* following them in a specific situation would be more dangerous than taking another course of action. For example, if a person has retreated to a locked room to protect him- or herself from a gunman in accordance with the company's plans, and the aggressor begins forcing the door open, it would likely be safer to climb out of a ground floor window than to remain in that room. After the explosion at Charlton County High School, the staff member who told the school administrator to completely change the response for the entire school must have felt empowered to give such advice. And when the administrator followed the directions of a subordinate, an even higher level of empowerment was demonstrated.

For someone who has never worked in a K–12 school, the level of empowerment and trust demonstrated by this incident might not be readily apparent. Later school crises have shown this is the exception, not the rule. Even today, there are still many schools where only the principal or headmaster can order a lockdown or authorize that 911 be called. Last year, our analysts learned that a school district with more than 100 schools had blocked the ability for staff to call 911 from most of the telephones in one of its high schools. This was apparently done to prevent staff from overreacting by calling 911 when it was not necessary. This example shows how easy it can be for an organization to fail to properly consider the need to adequately train staff so they can be trusted with the level of empowerment required to save lives in an emergency.

The dynamics of an organization can easily contribute to this. For example, the administrator of a school is the person who is ultimately held accountable for anything that goes wrong in the school. School principals can sometimes lose their position over a single crisis event. This helps us to understand how a decision could be made to deny staff the ability to call 911, even in a large school system. This dynamic can also easily result in a situation where micromanagement hinders crisis response during life and death incidents.

These types of cultural dynamics can be incredibly debilitating. One of the coauthors was conducting crisis simulations as part of a school safety, security, climate, culture, and emergency preparedness audit for a large urban school system in a community with a high rate of violence and gang activity. One of the test subjects was a school administrator who had been awarded the Bronze Star while serving as an officer in a combat unit with the U.S. Army a few years prior to the assessment. We would ordinarily anticipate that this individual would score very well on crisis simulations because he had experienced far more challenging situations than those depicted in even the most difficult scenarios we present. Surprisingly, the administrator's performance was far below average, and he repeatedly responded to scenarios by saying he would have to call the school district office for guidance.

After the assessment, the administrator remarked that the superintendent had been known to fire administrators for problems that went beyond the building level and that he and his colleagues were operating in an extremely unpredictable environment. The district was also experiencing an unusually high level of turnover among administrators and teachers. Our assessment revealed that his comments were not unique among test subjects. Observing an individual who could perform at such high levels in combat who had been rendered incapable of handling relatively minor school crisis scenarios was an eye-opening experience. Our report of findings recommended significant changes in empowerment and accountability, which were later implemented in the district.

This type of situation is not unique to schools. Leaders in other sectors may also have valid concerns that a staff member may overreact and evacuate or lock down a building when it is not appropriate. At the same time, all leaders must understand that mass casualty loss of human life can occur if they do not properly empower their personnel. While the culture of an organization can impact our ability to make decisions under stress, the structure of emergency plans and procedures can also create unintended obstacles.

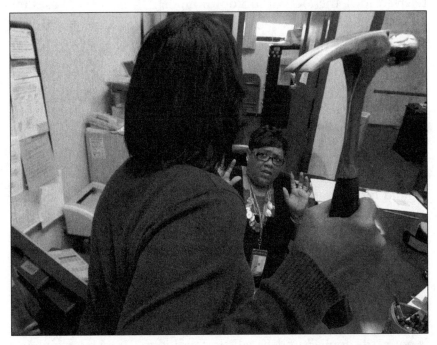

Scenario: Scenario-based training can prepare you for crisis situations through stress inoculation and the creation of a mental library of responses. This still from a school scenario-based training video reminds staff that guns are not the only items that can be used as weapons. The brutal murder of a Massachusetts schoolteacher by a student armed with a box cutter in October 2013 is a tragic illustration that there are many types of weapons used by aggressors.
Photo: Rachel Wilson

Structural Barriers to Effective Life and Death Decision Making

Evaluating emergency preparedness on a regular basis, we routinely see examples of crisis preparedness plan structures with significant barriers to life and death decision making. Though typically the result of well-intentioned efforts, these structural problems can overwhelm even the most dedicated and talented people in a crisis.

These procedures often sound logical until they are tested in a realistic manner that simulates stressful field conditions.

One example is an alternative approach to lockdowns for schools referred to as the lockout/lockdown model. This concept bases the type of lockdown on the location of the incident rather than the type and severity of the threat prompting a lockdown. For lockout, the assumption is that the potential danger exists outside the building. Typically, the exterior doors of the building are locked but interior doors such as classrooms, cafeterias, the main office, and media center doors are not locked, and movement of people is not restricted inside the school. In the lockout/lockdown approach, a lockdown is used if there is a threat inside the school. This concept has been around for more than a decade and is popular with many schools. This is because school administrators naturally do not like to shut down a school needlessly.

The problem is that we have found that this concept has a fail rate above 90 percent when tested by crisis simulations. This means that in schools that use this concept, staff typically do not think of a lockdown when it is an appropriate response. This is because the concept is not easily applied under realistic conditions. Though lockout and lockdown drills may go well, our experience has been that school employees presented with a variety of situations are unable to find an appropriate solution for scenarios that occur inside the school that do not involve someone brandishing a weapon. For example, when posed with scenarios depicting aggressive and emotionally unstable people, school employees often feel that locking down the entire school would be an overreaction. At the same time, the lockout option is useless because the aggressor is already inside the school and implementing a lockout will not protect anyone.

Another serious flaw with the lockout concept is that if a school implements a lockout due to a report of a potentially dangerous person outside the school, the person may gain access between the time the sighting is made and the lockout is implemented. It can be far more practical to use a planning strategy that includes a preventive lockdown option—often referred to as a soft lockdown—with the option to escalate to an emergency lockdown. With this approach, a preventive lockdown requires interior doors to be locked and movement in hallways to be restricted while the situation is evaluated but teaching and work activities continue.

For example, if an intoxicated and angry parent curses out school staff in the front office, the rest of the school interior can be secured while the police respond. If the person becomes physically violent, he or she will not have access to students and staff throughout the school. This is a very common occurrence for many schools, one that happens with much more frequency than an active shooter event. For more dire situations, the emergency lockdown is used, and all teaching and work activities cease while law enforcement officers respond. Students and school employees have been seriously injured and killed in situations that have not been properly contained before they escalated.

It is helpful to understand that both public and nonpublic schools experience situations where people who are intoxicated, emotionally unstable, and/or angry create a problem. School officials have in many instances underreacted to these situations because they have experience in handling what they feel are similar situations. There are still many schools in America where school officials will not call the police if a parent aggressively curses out staff in the presence of school children. A number of these situations have resulted in serious injury to staff and students. It is critical to remember that such persons may be armed. In some cases, students and staff have been killed because of this type of underreaction when this has turned out to be the case.

Whether you work in a factory, a department store, a government building, or a school, an underreaction like this can turn a relatively unpleasant encounter into a deadly one. As author and New York University professor Joe LeDoux puts it, "the cost of treating a stick as a snake is less than that of treating a snake as a stick," if you are hiking in the woods (Sherwood, 2010). Even though our society has loosened the definition of what is considered inappropriate behavior, it is important to remember that socially unacceptable patterns of behavior can be a significant warning sign of danger when violence is involved.

People who exhibit these and other warning signs like we discussed in Chapter Five are sending a clear signal that they do not understand or respect appropriate social behavior—at least at the moment. It is also critical to evaluate the situation within the proper context.

While some behaviors may border on inappropriate in a nightclub, they take on an even more significant meaning at work, in a place of worship, or in a school. When you see or hear the types of warning signs that de Becker identified, or any of the imminent warning signs of at-risk youth, think about them in the context of the Window of Life. For example, you should immediately consider where you can secure yourself, how you can protect others, how to evacuate the area, and how to quickly call for help as appropriate.

As an example, we teach schools to train and empower all employees to implement a preventive lockdown and call for law enforcement assistance whenever a visitor does any of the following in a school:

- yells, screams, or curses out an employee or student;
- makes any form of aggressive physical contact, like grabbing someone by the shirt collar;
- makes any statements threatening physical harm;
- deliberately breaches access control/visitor management policies; or
- forces an employee to clearly react to a situation as if he or she feels physically threatened.

These types of behaviors are often observed before a person becomes violent. In many cases, this type of behavior is exhibited just prior to an aggressor pulling and using a weapon. Underreaction in these types of circumstances can be deadly.

Reasonable guidance, structure, and support can unleash our incredible power to think and act appropriately, even under stressful and challenging situations. By looking at decades of research, evaluation, and assessment relating to how people make decisions under life and death conditions, you can prepare yourself to perform at impressive levels.

As with many of the concepts we have discussed, we should not assume that we will act logically while under extreme stress. As Grossman points out, the effects of combat stress are highly toxic and corrosive for human beings (Grossman and Christensen, 2011). We must understand that some incidents of violence are, in reality, forms of mortal combat between people. Few would argue that a police officer in a gunfight is in combat. A person who is being hunted by a gunman in a mall, factory, school, or office complex will also be under the tremendous and toxic stress of combat. Making a conscious decision to give yourself permission to live is one important way to help counter these corrosive effects. We can mentally and physically prepare ourselves for this. According to Grossman, the properly prepared human mind can be one of the most powerful survival tools available to us.

Conclusion

By developing a positive survival mindset and consciously making a decision to do everything within your power to survive, you are more likely to survive any deadly encounter where there is a window of opportunity to stay alive. Of course, there are limits to any strategy. Even the most elite soldiers are sometimes killed in combat. At the same time, when we examine how Navy SEAL Marcus Lutrell survived a major assault in Afghanistan in Chapter Twelve, we will see just how well developed the survival mechanisms of the modern soldier have become. Lutrell survived his incredible ordeal in part because he believed that he could. The decision to use your brain to survive no matter what it takes can mean the difference between life and death (Luttrell and Robinson, 2007). Going back to the explosion at Charlton County High School, imagine the stress that the school staff must have felt just after the blast. In a *New York Times* article about the incident, Dr. David Vukich from the University Medical Center in Jacksonville, Florida, said, "This is not the sort of thing you'd see on the streets of America . . . These are very serious, devastating military-type injuries," (12 students hurt, 1994). Just like those school staff overcame such a horrific event, you can improve the chances that you will succeed in almost any situation where survival is an option.

Key Points in Chapter Ten

- In a crisis, remember the Window of Life. Even the most effective actions may be useless if they are just a few seconds too late. This Window of Life can be a mere two seconds, or it can be longer.
- Even if an armed officer is in the facility, it can sometimes take one or more minutes for an officer to reach the location of the incident.
- The longer the delay in making the necessary decisions, the less chance you have to save lives or reduce the negative impact of an incident.
- Protect yourself first so you can more effectively protect others.
- Your odds of survival will go up if you take immediate action to prevent imminent harm before calling 911—unless you can do both at the same time.
- As a human being and a survivor, you are empowered not only to make decisions to save human lives but also to deviate from established plans and procedures to do so.
- All leaders must understand that mass casualty loss of human life can occur if they do not properly empower their personnel.
- Socially unacceptable patterns of behavior can be a significant warning sign of danger when violence is involved.
- As soon as you detect warning signs, consider where you can secure yourself, how you can protect others, how to evacuate the area, and how to quickly call for help as appropriate.

BIBLIOGRAPHY

12 students hurt when bazooka shell explodes. (1994). *The New York Times.* Retrieved from *http://www.nytimes.com/1994/11/04/us/12-students-hurt-when-bazooka-shell-explodes.html*

Dorn, M. (2012). Safe topics: The first 30 seconds. *Safe Topics.* Safe Havens International.

Grossman, D. and L. W. Christensen. (2011). *On combat: The psychology and physiology of deadly conflict in war and peace.* Milstadt, IL: Warrior Science Publications.

Luttrell, M., and P. Robinson. (2007). *Lone survivor: The eyewitness account of Operation Redwing and the lost heroes of SEAL Team 10.* Macon, GA: Boston: Little, Brown.

Sherwood, B. (2010). *The survivor's club: The secrets and science that could save your life.* New York: Grand Central Publishing.

CHAPTER ELEVEN

SATISFICING

This is another key to faster and more accurate decision making.

Today was the day. He was tired of hurting, and he was tired of the nightmare he had been born into. After hurting for so long, he had decided to end it. He sat in his bed, mentally reviewing his plans. Taking a deep breath, he took his .22 caliber pistol and went into his grandfather's room.

His grandfather was asleep in his bed, snoring softly. The boy stared at him for a moment, raised the pistol, and shot him twice in the head, then ten times in his chest. As he headed down the stairs he ran into his grandfather's girlfriend who was carrying a basket of laundry. Without a word he shot her twice in the head, watched her body roll down the stairs, picked his way through the fallen laundry, stepped over her body, and then headed outside (Hammers, 2007).

At 2:45 P.M., he drove his grandfather's squad car up to the doors at the front of Red Lake High School and got out wearing his grandfather's body armor and gun belt while brandishing his police tactical shotgun. Seeing the boy and sensing danger, the two unarmed security officers at the walk-through metal detector reacted immediately. One officer rapidly took refuge and survived the attack. The other bravely tried to stop the gunman, but the attempt failed as it only took a matter of seconds for the boy to aim and fire the shotgun, killing the dedicated officer (Alert system fell, 2005).

The deafening boom of the shotgun terrified a teacher in the hallway. The boy recognized her as one of his former teachers; he raised the shotgun and took a shot at her, missing. She ran into her classroom and locked the door (Maag, 2005).

He forced his way into the classroom by shooting out a large window alongside the door and stepping through. Once inside, he began methodically executing the teacher and the students. The only time he was interrupted was when a student lunged at him and stabbed him with a pencil. But this student's heroic efforts were also ineffective, and he was shot three times.

The bodies of the teacher and her students lay a short distance from a second door to the classroom. This door could have provided an escape route for the victims had this option been selected in time. But this ruthless attack happened fast—very fast. The killer would inflict the most damage in the first 90 seconds or so of what would end up being an extraordinarily long school shooting incident.

The students and teacher who died were obviously under pressure to make a series of high-stakes decisions. They had limited information available to them since the front office had issued no instructions. These decisions had to be made in an extremely limited window of time and under the threat of imminent death. The pressure was immense. Unfortunately, like the victims of the Our Lady of Angels fire, they had been inadvertently trained to die.

Tribal police officers arrived quickly and engaged the killer in a gun battle. Fortunately, the officers were armed with tactical rifles, and they were able to wound the aggressor. After an eight-minute killing spree that left ten students dead, the killer committed suicide.

The school district settled all 26 lawsuits filed against it. Shortly after the case was settled, plaintiff's attorneys asked two experts from different firms to conduct double-blind evaluations to assess the work of a school safety-consulting firm that had worked extensively to prepare students and staff at the school for emergencies. The firm and school had focused specifically on active shooter incidents, and numerous drills had been conducted at the school. According to the massive case file sent to coauthor Michael Dorn, who was one of the expert witnesses selected for the case, this terrible attack occurred with such speed and intensity that no one in the office ever announced a lockdown. In addition, the case file indicates that the school's crisis plans had been developed in a manner that not only failed to empower staff to make independent decisions but, even worse, implied that they could not. This can seriously degrade the ability of people to adjust to fit a specific incident. For example, the written plans did not provide the empowerment needed for staff to be able to make the connection that they could to evacuate a room during a lockdown.

Victims of violent incidents often lack the time to think and make decisions before taking action. In order to survive, victims often have to act very fast. So what should you do to prepare to think and act fast?

The Concept of Satisficing

The approaches outlined in previous chapters would have likely improved the odds of survival in this situation. However, the relevant point for this chapter is the speed with which people must make decisions and take action for chaotic and fast-breaking situations. As we have pointed out, people who have never been shot at or otherwise violently attacked often have difficulty comprehending just how fast violent encounters can occur. The perceptions of most people regarding acts of violence are sometimes based on limited personal experience and, more typically, on what they see depicted on television and in movies. This can lead to a disconnect between expectations and reality when witnessing acts of unbridled aggression.

In a school shooting, there are often delays ranging from one to eight minutes from the time shots are fired until the time the office orders a lockdown. The concepts we have already covered help to explain several of the reasons for these types of critical and potentially deadly delays. When faced with an attack like the one that took place at the Red Lake Reservation School, this tendency can result in deadly delays. The same dynamic can be seen in more typical single-victim attacks. This is because trying to find a perfect response to the assault will typically have one or both of the following outcomes:

(1) the reaction will be too slow to be effective, and (2) the actions taken will be less effective than those taken reflexively.

In his excellent book *Sources of Power: How People Make Decisions,* Dr. Gary Klein (1998) explains that we are capable of making effective decisions in what at first appear to be almost "no-win" situations. Klein describes how a strategy called "recognition-primed decision making" allows people with a high level of experience to see a crisis situation for what it is so they are able not only to resolve it sooner but also to do so in a highly skilled manner. Klein explains that by moving in the right direction intuitively and without taking the precious time to compare one option against another, we can increase performance because that approach fits with the way our brain works under such conditions. Klein found that even though we have just developed a new course of action for a unique scenario, this approach could be quite effective (Klein, 1998).

Klein also describes a concept developed by Nobel Prize winner Herbert Simon called "satisficing." According to Simon, satisficing is choosing the first option that appears likely to work based on the situation rather than trying to overanalyze each option (Simon, 1956). Though it is a relatively simple concept, it can be among one of the most important aspects of life and death decision making for you to understand. It can also be among the most difficult for us to accept on an emotional level. We have found that this approach can help you understand ways to better address some of the more complex and challenging crisis situations you may face.

On the other hand, when people try to find an optimal solution to a serious problem, it can be less effective. Klein calls this approach "optimizing." Optimizing asks that we seek more information and reason through the problem so that we can make the best decision. Some salient examples of optimizing are the processes of purchasing a car, accepting a new job, or trimming our family budget. While this approach may work well when we have plenty of time to obtain more information and consider the advantages and disadvantages of each, crisis situations do not afford us this luxury.

Like many victims of violent crime, the teachers and students at Red Lake were not able to learn more about what was happening. They also did not have much time to analyze this limited information. In many crisis situations, the likely outcome of the event is, to an extent, predetermined rather than decided on the day of the incident. For example, the crisis plan written for the school by the consulting firm was not based on the types of research we have discussed in this book. In fact, the plans were developed in ways that typically result in exactly the type of catastrophic plan failure that occurred that day. And when the plans were drilled to reinforce the way they were written, students and staff were literally drilled to die.

The school's crisis plans were developed in a manner that prohibited rather than instilled independent thought and action. For example, the plans identified the action steps staff should take once the call for lockdown was announced, but the plans did not encourage—or even allow—staff to call for a lockdown. In addition, the last action step for the school's lockdown procedure was "STAY PUT!!" With the luxury of hindsight and a lack of imminent danger, it may be obvious to the reader that when the aggressor forced his way into one classroom, the best course of action would have been for all students and the teacher to flee out of a door in the back of the classroom rather than staying in the room as the plan directed.

As with the monthly fire drills conducted before the OLA fire, Red Lake staff were not required to make the independent decision to implement a lockdown during drills. Instead, like the majority of K–12 schools in America today, drills were conducted in a top-down fashion that did not properly prepare students and staff to deviate from plans if the need to do so should arise. Grossman explains how powerfully destructive these types of practices can be with a story about a police officer who received training on how to take a handgun away from an aggressor. When the officer was trained, he was told that he would have to practice extensively to be able to perform it reliably under field conditions. He practiced this technique over and over with his wife using an unloaded handgun. He would disarm his wife, hand her the gun, and repeat the technique until he had truly mastered it. He became extremely proficient in disarming her. One evening, while on a call with another officer, the officer suddenly found himself confronted by a man who was pointing a handgun at him. Without hesitation, he did exactly as he had practiced countless times: he snatched the gun from the aggressor's hands, and much to the astonishment of all parties involved, he handed the gun back to the aggressor. The second officer was able to react quickly by shooting the aggressor, allowing the officer to survive this potentially deadly blunder.

The officer had inadvertently done exactly what the staff at the Our Lady of Angels School had done. He had programmed his brain the wrong way. This underscores the need for logical and proven approaches to training. Understanding satisficing and accepting that this is the most efficient way to make crisis decisions can help us avoid bad habits that can interfere with our amazingly capable brains.

The Power of Naturalistic Thinking

Klein identified a "singular evaluation" strategy as the primary approach that veteran firefighters used to make critical decisions under the pressure caused by limited information and timeframes (Klein, 1998). This means that the person does not compare options analytically like we might do when choosing where to go on vacation. Instead, our brains work quickly to choose the best logical path. By reacting in what he calls a naturalistic manner, we can make improved decisions faster so they are more likely to have a positive effect on the situation.

Klein describes naturalistic thinking as well suited for life and death situations. For example, if an airline pilot or military commander makes a mistake, several hundred or even thousands of people can perish. Even though a mistake by an attorney, engineer, or accountant can have far-reaching and severe life-altering consequences, they are not under the time constraints that a surgeon, police officer, or emergency medical technician faces.

Klein focused his research on what he calls "experienced decision makers." These are individuals, who, by nature of their training and work, have a considerable base of knowledge in making critical decisions that can have life and death consequences. For example, the fire commanders in one study his team conducted were found to have an average experience level of 23 years in the art of fighting fires and saving lives.

The Power of Operating from a Base of Knowledge

Klein concluded that our brains are very capable of making high-stakes decisions quickly and with a high degree of accuracy. This is true as long as we have what he calls a "base of knowledge." Our base of knowledge is created both through practical experience and through effective training that utilizes realistic simulations (Klein, 1998). Once we have a solid base of knowledge, our brains can work faster and more effectively to respond to challenging situations. This can also be affected by how we use simulations to prepare for life and death events. Grossman states that training that provides what he calls "stress inoculation" is how soldiers and police prepare for the severe stress of combat. He asserts that the more realistic training simulations are, the better prepared we will be. Controlled testing has indeed shown that when law enforcement officers can use regular practice and training to learn to function with a greatly reduced heart rate, performance is greatly improved (Grossman, 2011).

If the ability to evaluate an aggressor with a weapon and react is critical to an armed police officer, it can be even more important to the survival of an unarmed civilian facing the same threat. Though the officer is far more likely to encounter this type of situation, the unarmed civilian faced with this circumstance has a dire need to act immediately. Like the police officer, the civilian must recognize the situation and take instant action. Unlike the law enforcement professional, the unarmed civilian usually does not have a way of neutralizing the aggressor with any degree of reliability. Even a veteran martial artist cannot reliably neutralize a gunman in many situations.

The concepts we outlined earlier—pattern matching, mental simulation, and Dorn Drills—can dramatically increase the chances that you will be able to perform at this level. If you are mentally prepared to use satisficing and naturalistic thinking, your chances of survival are even better. These techniques help us prepare to act to save lives in a manner consistent with how our brains and bodies are supposed to work.

A secretary, tractor-trailer truck driver, construction worker, schoolteacher, minister, hairstylist, bartender, or CEO of a Fortune 500 company can easily improve his or her odds of surviving a deadly encounter. We cannot offer you any assurances that you will survive, but your chances of surviving those incidents where a Window of Life exists can be raised dramatically with these proven approaches.

By practicing for challenging scenarios and simulating a response using satisficing, you can train your brain to engage more rapidly. This can help you internalize the approach of shifting from traditional decision making for routine tasks to the approach used to make high-stakes decisions under extreme time pressure. Though it fits with how our brains work under life and death situations, making satisficing a conditioned response will take additional practice. Doing so will pay dividends when you have other important decisions to make, even if they are not of a life and death nature. Like pattern matching, satisficing can improve your quality of life even if you are fortunate enough to never face a life-threatening situation.

Conclusion

When we consider our awesome power to save human lives, we can only wonder how many more people would be saved in deadly encounters if more people knew about these skills. Proper life and death decisions are being made every day using these techniques. People who face death are safely reunited with loved ones each day because of the decisions of those who are properly prepared to take immediate life-saving action. The actions that will need to be taken will vary widely and can differ dramatically in two seemingly identical scenarios. Understanding and trusting our ability to make rapid decisions more effectively can be more critical than how well we can follow a specific plan.

Returning to the deadly Red Lake attack may help illustrate this point. There is no lockdown protocol that will be perfect for every possible school shooting. Action steps that would have worked extremely well for the Columbine High School attack were not effective for this situation because of one difference—the attacker decided to force his way into individual classrooms to kill. The basic differences in the design of these two schools also illustrates why one lockdown plan cannot be used safely for all schools. Perhaps more importantly, our ability to rapidly deviate from emergency procedures without taking the time to ask a supervisor for permission can be incredibly important.

In this case, a schoolteacher was faced with an aggressor with two highly lethal police firearms. By the time she encountered him, he already had experience killing with both of the weapons. The aggressor forced his way into her classroom and began shooting. A valiant attempt by an unarmed security officer to attack the gunman had also been in vain, costing the shooter only one round of ammunition and a few seconds of his time, but at the cost of one precious human life. A student was also shot when he attempted to attack the killer with an improvised weapon. In an armed attack, there is no "time out" or automatic replay. The only time that matters is the time we have to act based on the situation and the information we have available in the first few seconds of a crisis. As this case illustrates, whether the action is to lock a door to keep a gunman out or to evacuate a classroom full of students when a gunman is forcing his way into the room, actions that are intended to avoid death must usually be made in seconds rather than minutes. Satisficing can help us make these types of decisions more effectively and quickly so our actions matter when lives hang in the balance.

Key Points in Chapter Eleven

- Victims of violent incidents often lack the time to stop and think before making decisions and taking action.
- Satisficing is choosing the first option that appears likely to work based on the situation rather than trying to overanalyze each option.
- Optimizing works best with time to obtain information. Sometimes in a crisis you do not have time to optimize your decisions and can only do what time allows.
- Our base of knowledge is created through practical experience and effective training.
- The more realistic training simulations are, the better prepared we will be.
- By practicing for challenging scenarios and simulating a response using satisficing, you can train your brain to engage more rapidly in a crisis.
- Be careful not to accidentally create deadly habits when you practice for emergencies.

BIBLIOGRAPHY

Alert system fell silent during Red Lake school shooting. (2005). PostBulletin.com. Retrieved from *http://www.postbulletin.com/alert-system-fell-silent-during-red-lake-school-shooting/article_8d3095d4-38a7-58b8-84f0-4e659f963f56.html?mode=jqm*

Grossman, D. and L. W. Christensen. (2011). *On combat: The psychology and physiology of deadly conflict in war and peace.* Milstadt, IL: Warrior Science Publications.

Hammers, D. (2007). Second victim known as more than footnote: Michelle Sigana left behind a loving family that remembers her generosity. Pioneer Press. Retrieved from *http://www.highbeam.com/doc/1G1-143485591.html*

Klein, G. (1998). *Sources of power: How people make decisions.* Cambridge, MA: The MIT Press.

Maag, C. (2005). The devil in Red Lake. *Time* Magazine. Retrieved from *http://www.time.com/time/subscriber/article/0,33009,1042470-4,00.html*

Simon, H. A. (1956). Rational choice and the structure of the environment. *Psychological Review, 63,* 129–138.

CHAPTER TWELVE

ACTIVE SHOOTERS— SHOULD YOU RUN, HIDE, OR FIGHT?

Training people to attack an active shooter as a last resort without an adequate scope of scenarios can result in unexpected stress reactions.

William McMullen was excited. It wasn't that he was in the Iroquois Theater, the newest theater in Chicago, or that the famous Eddie Foy was here for the current burlesque, *Mr. Bluebeard*. William was excited because after several days of sparse crowds, the Iroquois was packed to the rafters with men, women, and children who had come for the matinee. The laughter of the crowd through the first act made up for the poor crowds of the past few days and the cold weather outside.

William proudly looked around at the Iroquois. It was six magnificent stories of marble columns and mahogany accents. He was proud to be employed in a modern and safe theater. When he was hired, his boss had showed him how the Iroquois was "absolutely fireproof," including the new asbestos curtain that could be lowered to separate the audience from any fire on the stage.

All of that disappeared as the pit orchestra started playing "In the Pale Moonlight" at the start of Act II. From his vantage point above the stage, William watched the stage curtain being drawn. His excitement turned to shock as he saw the curtain brush up against the back of a spotlight and burst into flame. He reached out in an attempt to put the fire out, but the curtain was just beyond his reach, and the fire began to spread. William scrambled down the scaffolding and grabbed the on-duty fireman. He pointed up and whispered, "Fire!"

The fireman's eyes widened, and his breath fluffed up his beard and moustache. Without another sound, he grabbed a Kilfyres fire extinguisher and clambered up the ladder. The powder-based extinguisher was no match for the blaze. The fireman began climbing down and called out, loud enough to be heard in the first few rows of the audience, "I can't stop it!"

Eddie Foy pointed at William and called out, "Lower the fire curtain!"

As William pulled the rope to lower the curtain, Foy stepped out by the footlights and spoke to the crowd, "Ladies and gentlemen! Please remain calm! Everything is under control!"

As if to solidify the irony, several things happened at once—a common theme in disasters. The asbestos curtain caught on a light, leaving several feet between the bottom of the curtain and the stage; a piece of burning debris fell at Eddie Foy's feet, causing the audience to stagger backward in fright, and the actors and actresses fled out of a door in the rear of the theater.

When the rear door opened, cold air rushed in, feeding the fire on the stage and causing a huge fireball to erupt. This fireball rushed under the asbestos curtain and reached all the way up to the balconies, igniting everything flammable along the way. The audience, already panicked by the small flame that had fallen on Foy, now stampeded toward the exits.

William stood, transfixed, watching the audience's transformation from a happy crowd into a senseless mob. Men and women pushed children out of the way and everyone rushed the doors. Several of the exits had locked iron gates. A few of the doors that the crowd ran to were actually locked windows that had been painted to look like doors. Still others had a new, confusing type of handle, and most of the others opened inward. As we have seen in many other disasters over the past century, the people in front were crushed, and the people in back kept pushing. After a few seconds, people began climbing over bodies toward the exits. All around was the sound of wailing and screaming and the crack of broken bones. William stood listening, tears streaming down his face as he watched people who were about to die by the hundreds. He was only jarred back to the reality by the sudden jarring sensation of Eddie Foy grabbing his arm and yelling, "We gotta go!"

The Iroquois Theater fire was the most lethal theater fire in U.S. history. The dead were reportedly stacked ten high in some of the exits. Others jumped from high windows, with the first few dying, but providing a cushion for those who jumped after them. More than 575 people died, with more than 30 dying later in hospitals. Exact numbers could not be calculated because numerous burned bodies were moved to accommodate the fire response (Iroquois Theater, 2007).

This story is one of numerous examples studied by fire service professionals and experts in crowd behavior to help us understand how people in crowds who are in fear for their lives can act. These incidents have revealed that when people run to escape an enclosed area, they can block exit doors, slowing evacuation and causing mass casualty loss of human life. Amanda Ripley provides numerous compelling examples of the risk of a stampede during a disaster in her book *The Unthinkable: Who Survives When Disasters Strike and Why*. As she phrases it, "faster is slower" can be the case in many emergencies (Ripley, 2008).

What If He Had Really Been a Killer?

In early 2013 and in the wake of the Sandy Hook tragedy, an Iowa high school student spotted a man who was wearing a handgun in a holster walking in the hallway of her school. She immediately entered a classroom and told her teacher what she had seen. Initially, the teacher thought she was joking, but finally the student was able to convince the teacher that there really was a man with a gun in the school.

Having recently completed a popular live training program where she was taught to attack an active shooter as a last resort, the teacher prepared to fight back. She instructed her students to prepare to throw books at the man if he entered the classroom. The teacher then grabbed a fire extinguisher, steeling herself to do battle with a gunman. However, the man turned out to be a fire marshal and was not there to attack anyone. Once the facts were known, the teacher's actions were reviewed to see how the concepts she had been taught had worked. This revealed that the approach would have likely increased the chances of death and serious injury at the school had the man actually been there to carry out a mass casualty shooting.

This story was shared with us by a colleague who is a school security professional with more than 25 years of experience working with schools across the country. In his view, there were significant concerns with the teacher's response. He points out that the teacher became so focused on attacking the "gunman" as a first option instead of as a last resort that she forgot to perform several critical action steps to protect herself, her students, and the rest of the school. For example, the teacher failed to remember to:

1. close the classroom door,
2. lock the classroom door,
3. call the office so the office could in turn order a lockdown, and
4. call 911.

This incident reinforces our skepticism regarding such approaches. His concerns—and those of many other professionals and public safety officials—is that some approaches to training school employees to attack an active shooter may actually increase danger in certain situations.

Fighting for Life

Jacob Ryker reacted well under pressure. He had been shot in the chest, but he was still able to jump onto the student who had been firing a .22 caliber semiautomatic rifle in his school's cafeteria. Seizing the opportunity, and with help from his younger brother and another student, Jacob was able to subdue the shooter and successfully end the attack.

Although two people died from their wounds, and another 21 people besides Jacob were wounded, the shooter would never have a chance to fire the more than 600 rounds of remaining ammunition he had with him because of Jacob's actions. When the students attacked the shooter, they stopped the violent rampage and changed the outcome of the terrible incident. No one had ever taught them to do this—they just knew it needed to be done, and they acted (Longman, 1998). As illustrated by this example and several others, there is evidence that unarmed people can sometimes stop a person with a gun if conditions are right.

As illustrated from these stories, the options of running, hiding, or fighting during an active shooter incident can be either an effective or a deadly choice. So which, if any, of these options should you choose if you see someone with a weapon or hear gunfire? This chapter is focused on providing you with helpful information on these and other options. Our goal is to help you better understand these concepts and when to apply them—or not.

Should You Run?

Shortly after the shooting at a movie theater in Aurora, Colorado, the Houston, Texas, Police Department released a video called *Run, Hide, Fight: Surviving an Active Shooter Event* that they had produced with grant funding from the U.S. Department of Homeland Security. The video was produced on a compressed schedule due to the timely nature of the information after the shooting in Aurora (Controversial city, 2012). The video's release was widely covered by the media and millions of people have viewed it. The video instructs viewers that they have three options if faced with an active shooter situation. The video states that the first option is, "If you can get out, do" (Ready Houston, 2012). But is running from an active shooter really the fastest way to get to safety?

Suppose you were in a building and heard gunshots, but you did not know where the gunman or gunmen were. Should you run, or would it be safer to secure yourself in a lockable space? People have been shot when they were trying to escape in this manner before. This happened in the cafeteria at Columbine High School where students who attempted to run from the killers were also murdered (Cullen, 2009). However, no student or employee who was in a locked room was killed during the lengthy attack in 1999.

Is it wise for an elementary teacher to evacuate students from a classroom when there is an active shooter in the school? Actual shooting incidents can be very confusing, and survivors often relate that they were unable to tell exactly where gunfire was coming from. Many practitioners are especially concerned about the idea of asking pre-K students, persons with special needs, hospital patients, and the elderly to attempt to outrun a gunman. For example, it is clear from information that has been confirmed at the point of this writing that the tragedy at Sandy Hook Elementary School would have been even more catastrophic if all teachers had evacuated their classrooms upon hearing the first gunshots.

Since the release of the *Run, Hide, Fight* video, officials from many school districts and independent schools have been advised by law enforcement to use this video for staff training and, in some instances, to train students. It is very important to note that in at least two instances that we are aware of, local police have instructed school districts to discontinue the use of all other plan components and replace them with this video. This is particularly disturbing because even if all of the instructions in this video were sound and appropriate for all situations and environments, the video contains no information at all pertaining to fires, tornadoes, earthquakes, accidents, medical emergencies, or any type of weapons situation other than an active shooter. As these other incidents represent the vast majority of all deaths on school property, it is illogical and dangerous to disregard all other hazards and focus only on active shooter situations. This recommendation would also probably increase civil liability in the event of a death or injury in a school where this approach was applied.

We also see a few other potentially dangerous instructions in the video. Since it places running as the first option, it means that evacuation is always to be used first in contrast to a lockdown. The video repeatedly tells the viewers that their first option in a shooting is to run. But is this always a sound approach?

One of the main concerns voiced by advocates of the Run, Hide, Fight approach is that the traditional lockdown concept has failed. Advocates of this position maintain that victims have been left in vulnerable positions by being trapped in rooms where they were killed because they had been conditioned to "cower in the dark" and wait helplessly for police to arrive. However, there has only been one incident in an educational facility that we are currently aware of where a gunman breached a locked classroom door and murdered multiple victims. The only incident of this type at a school that we are familiar with is the Red Lake School shooting described earlier. As previously noted, there were significant issues with the school's planning and drill program when it came to lockdowns. We should also point out that the use of the traditional lockdown approach was not a basis for the civil actions that followed the shooting.

While there are clearly issues with the way some organizations apply lockdown concepts, it is illogical to completely disregard the benefits of a proven method and replace it with an approach—running—that has not yet been validated and has been known to result in mass casualty deaths and injuries in some situations. One concern we have is that teaching people to run is further complicating a difficult concept while ignoring the opportunities to enhance current approaches. For example, running as a first option in an active shooter situation could cause catastrophic loss of life in a number of specific settings including:

- daycare centers,
- K–12 schools, facilities serving pre-K, kindergarten, and lower grade students and/or students with special needs,
- places of worship with childcare and youth programs,

- hospitals,
- rest homes, and
- mental heath facilities.

Of particular concern to us are the reactions we have seen from a number of school employees we have interviewed after they have seen this video. They have often told us that they would instruct their students to immediately run from the school if they hear gunfire—even if they do not know where it is coming from. When we seek clarification, they frequently tell us that they would evacuate their classrooms even when they have concrete block walls and solid wood doors with a sturdy lock. These same school staff also indicated that they would evacuate even if they knew the gunfire was coming from outside of the school and they were inside the building. Take a moment to imagine this scenario in a school with 2,000 high school students and an active shooter roaming the halls or a shootout between rival gang members near a school.

While viewers are cautioned that they should run "when it is safe to do so," they are told this while the video depicts people running. This is an important point because with this style of depiction, viewers tend to recall what they see rather than what they are told (Medina, 2009). The video then tells viewers repeatedly to run as their first option without this caution. Regardless of the intended message, some school employees only retain the idea that they should evacuate anytime they hear gunfire.

Experts have expressed two concerns on this point. The first is that teaching people to run, especially with a dramatic video, could result in a stampede. As numerous people have been killed in this manner already, we feel this concern bears careful consideration. Second, there is considerable evidence that running slows evacuation times when people are in any location with limited exit points due to the jamming of people in choke points such as exit doorways as described earlier.

Gregory Thomas is one of the nation's most respected and trusted school safety experts. He was selected as the lead author for a series of books on school safety published by Jane's, the go-to publisher for military and government security officials. Thomas has worked on numerous projects for federal agencies including the U.S. Departments of Education and Homeland Security. Thomas is also a former assistant commissioner for public safety education for the New York City Fire Department and served as the executive director of the Office of School Safety and Planning for the New York City Schools for many years. Like most school safety experts with extensive national experience, he is highly skeptical of the Run, Hide, Fight concept and other approaches that teach people to attack an active shooter in the school setting. He points out that "run" is in stark opposition to what research shows us about people running.

Amanda Ripley explains this concern with what experts call the "faster is slower effect." She points out that researchers have documented that people who rush for exits often jam up in doorways and other restricted areas, causing delays in trying to escape (Ripley, 2008). If enough people are present, these delays could be truly catastrophic as people pile up in exit ways. As Thomas points out, whether the threat is fire or a firearm, people exposed to danger will usually experience fear. Essentially, teaching people to "run" may cause mass casualty loss of life just like we described in the Iroquois Theater fire example and many other examples throughout history.

So When Could Run Be a Viable Option?

Although running from an armed attacker on open ground with no obstructions may be prudent, running inside a building could slow your escape and reduce your chances of survivability. The Clark County School District in Las Vegas, Nevada, has carefully studied the movement of large groups of students in an emergency. By videotaping and evaluating emergency drills at hundreds of schools, they have found that large groups of students can be evacuated much faster using a series of relatively simple techniques.

One of the most important techniques is the fast walk. Through measurement and independent evaluation of individual school evacuations, the Student Safety and Threat Evaluation Team found that evacuation time could be reduced by 30 percent. By testing their concepts with actual time and properly evaluated evacuation drills, they developed one of the most cutting-edge life-saving concepts available to schools today. Students are taught to run if they are exposed to gunfire while outdoors in an open area; however, students and staff are trained and drilled not to run but instead to move briskly and with purpose to escape from other types of danger—reducing the chances that people will be trampled.

Another concept that many experts find to be troubling is training people to run in a zigzag fashion if they are being shot at. Greg Elefritz, an Ohio police officer and president of Active Response Training, is among the experts who have questioned the validity of this concept. Conducting a series of simulations using paintball rounds and role players, he found that a gunman actually has a higher hit rate when victims try to flee in this fashion. Role players who ran in a straight line were hit less frequently, with fewer serious injuries. In addition, Elefritz found that people fell more often when trying to run in a zigzag pattern. Even though Elefritz cautions that these simulations were not scientifically conducted, they clearly raise concerns about the wisdom of training people in a concept that has not been proven to work in the civilian arena.

Should You Hide?

The lockdown technique has successfully protected staff and students in schools as far back as 1900. On May 12, 1900, a man named Herbert Horton came to a schoolhouse in Danbury, Connecticut, with a loaded revolver and demanded to see Lillian Owen, a teacher who he had been stalking. Miss Owen and her students barricaded the door, and Horton shot himself when he was unable to breach the door. This incident occurred just a few miles from the future site of Sandy Hook Elementary School (School teacher, 1900). Lockdown is a concept that has been successfully applied to protect students and staff for more than a century, with many other examples that have not made the national news because no lives were lost.

The traditional view has been that lockdown (i.e., hiding) is the best first option for many situations where there are indications that an aggressor with a weapon is nearby. While this approach has been, and should be, questioned and refined, we still feel that it should be the first course of action for situations where an armed aggressor is not yet in a confined space with potential victims and where lockable space is available. We have seen many instances where a promptly implemented lockdown prevented an active shooter from, accessing potential victims. For example, no staff or students died behind secured classroom doors in the Columbine, Virginia Tech, or Sandy Hook incidents. In the Virginia Tech shooting, students and staff in some rooms were able to barricade doors to their classrooms and survived. In the Sandy Hook incident, the killer attacked staff and students in the hallways and in two classrooms that were not locked. The main limitation for lockdown has been the ability of people to make the decision to use it and to act fast enough to implement it.

We feel this is particularly important when you do not know the location of an armed aggressor in or near a facility. As we mentioned previously, it can be very difficult to tell where the sound of gunfire is coming from during an attack. Considering that multiple people have been shot when they attempted to evacuate and encountered an active shooter, this technique has not been properly validated. This can be especially dangerous if there are multiple assailants and explosive devices, as was the case in the Columbine High School attack.

This danger can also be present in a terrorist attack. In a deadly attack at a boarding school in Nigeria on July 7, 2013, terrorists killed 27 students and staff by setting fire to a school and then shooting evacuees as they emerged (Ola, 2013). As shooters in the United States in at least four different school shootings have used similar tactics, this is not strictly a theoretical concern. In the recent terrorist attack at a shopping mall in Kenya, one survivor credited her escape with her decision to hide first and only run when the attack had subsided. "My instinct said, don't go with the crowd, move away from the crowd because the crowd is going to be the most vulnerable place." Elaine Dang eventually escaped after playing dead until the attackers had left the area and she saw other victims escaping safely (Kenya mall attack, 2013).

While evacuation is an option people should be trained in, there have often been large numbers of people who have successfully used the option to lockdown during active shooter incidents. Schools often use what is known as a "room clear" protocol to deal with specific evacuations. A room clear protocol is a simple procedure that allows any school employee to rapidly evacuate an area and move to safety in another location when there is danger. The room clear procedure provides a variation on a full-scale evacuation when that size of response would be detrimental. For example, if a person started shooting in a crowded cafeteria, the room clear protocol would be used to move students out of the cafeteria and to safety with two words, rather than an evacuation protocol that could also send more potential victims into danger as they leave classrooms.

In this type of situation, students are normally directed to a lockable area rather than evacuating. If a school has regular room clear drills, students and staff are more likely to act without being told to do so because they have been conditioned to react this way.

Our video unit helps schools develop custom training videos for these emergency protocols. This allows staff and students to train in the same proven way that airlines teach passengers what to do in an emergency. Commercial airlines do not make every passenger slide down an emergency chute for each flight, and for a variety of sound reasons. However, many school systems use a combination of short instructional videos combined with drills to teach students and staff how to perform functions like a lockdown, reverse evacuation, or room clear. These videos also instruct the viewer to be prepared to move from one protocol to another and to be ready to combine protocols as needed for specific situations. For example, a teacher who sees a gunman while outside at recess can use the reverse evacuation protocol to move students indoors quickly and then follow up with a lockdown protocol once inside. A planned school shooting was prevented in exactly this manner in Macon, Georgia, in September 2013. Increasingly, schools use custom web courses and videos to teach students and staff how to implement emergency procedures quickly for any type of situation.

Using these methods, people can be adequately prepared to respond to a broad array of situations without significant disruption to normal business. For example, our experience has been that the more schools focus on active shooter situations, the worse they will perform in an actual attack. Conducting a wider array of drills like fire, tornado, lockdown, room clear, reverse evacuation, and earthquake can help people better prepare to adapt rapidly to any situation they face. When combined with mental simulations and Dorn Drills, people can dramatically improve survivability for any type of incident with limited time investment on a day-to-day basis.

Should You Fight?

Does fighting an active shooter as a last resort reduce your chances of being killed? Our view is that it depends largely on what you are taught, how you are trained, and how much diversity is included in your scenario and mental simulation practice. The fight option is introduced as the third option in the *Run, Hide, Fight* video. It is also taught in several different training programs to employees and students at a number of K–12 schools, colleges, and universities.

While all of the coauthors are in agreement that it would sometimes be the best option for someone who is trapped in a room to fight an active shooter, we are deeply concerned about the way schools and other organizations are implementing these concepts. We are far from the only experts in the field who have expressed this concern. This is based on a careful review of the research on how people make life and death decisions as well as the sometimes astounding scenario responses we get from people who have been trained on this approach. Like most veteran law enforcement officers, coauthor Michael Dorn has also had firsthand experience in surviving multiple attacks by aggressors armed with guns, knives, and other weapons. Our concern is not focused on the concept of victims attacking an active shooter, but rather what we believe is the high degree of likelihood that people will misapply this tactic because of the way it is currently being presented.

The real-life example from the high school in Iowa where students spotted a potential gunman matches closely with what research and controlled simulations indicate are likely to occur when this approach is used. Our concern is that these techniques can sometimes be very difficult for laypeople to apply based on a short video or a 2-, 5-, or even 16-hour training program. The level of complexity of many of these techniques is better suited for a military special operator that has extensive training and a broad base of knowledge.

For example, the Heimlich maneuver is easily taught and applied because there are relatively few variables in how the technique can be applied. People who are choking to death act in fairly predictable ways. They are also not very likely to shoot at you, set off an explosive device, or attack you with a claw hammer. This makes it practical to teach people a series of simple and easy to understand action steps that often work very effectively to prevent death. The lives of thousands of people have been saved because they have seen a poster or completed training on this maneuver.

In contrast, teaching lifeguards to save people who are drowning is much more complex. People who are drowning sometimes overwhelm and drown those who are trying to rescue them. For this reason, the concepts taught to lifeguards are much more complicated than those for the Heimlich maneuver. As evidence of this, the American Red Cross Lifeguarding course takes at least twenty-five hours to complete. (Lifeguarding, 2013).

Can it really be easier to learn how to attack a determined aggressor who is firing a gun than to save a drowning person? Even though the concepts for responding to an armed aggressor might be read-ily applied by an experienced police officer or military veteran with combat experience, can the average department store manager, stockbroker, secretary, fifth grader, or college student realistically learn when it is appropriate to fight and how to do it with just a few hours or, in many cases, even minutes of training?

We propose that active shooter situations are even more complex and unpredictable than most situations a lifeguard might experience. For example, active shooter situations have sometimes involved the use of explosives, fire, and other weapons. Although people may be desperate for a simple solution, these solutions do not always exist. Our experience has been that the current methodologies for teaching people when they should and should not attack an active shooter are not adequate to convey the complexity of the concepts being taught. Law enforcement officers experience a wide array of scenarios to learn when and how to apply deadly force. In contrast, at the time of this writing, all of the training programs that teach people to fight back are focused almost exclusively on incidents involving guns.

Even though we have seen some thoughtfully delivered training for teachers on how to react to active shooters and even attack gun-men, the participants in our scenario simulation assessments who have completed this type of training focus on the fight aspect of the training. After receiving this type of training, school staff are typ-ically more likely to attack a person in any type of crisis situation, even ones where it would not make sense based on the situation and could even increase the chances of injury or loss of life with no real benefit to the safety of the overall school.

One basis for approaches where unarmed civilians are being taught to attack an active shooter relies on a version of distraction theory (VanMeenen, et al., 2006). This approach teaches people how to throw objects at a shooter's head to momentarily distract him, followed by a coordinated attack by multiple people in the room. At least two different training programs and a training video devel-oped by a university police department teach students in both K–12 schools and institutions of higher learning to throw books and other objects at a gunman while others fight the attacker. This approach has been among the most highly controversial, as students as young as kindergarteners have been taught these concepts (Students taught, 2008). This approach has been widely implemented in the People's Republic of China where at least one school official has already been stabbed to death while trying to follow this policy (Yao, 2013).

Other programs for schools emphasize that only employees should be taught to attack an active shooter and that it is clearly not appropriate to train K–12 students in these techniques. There has been a significant amount of debate on this point, even between proponents of these two different approaches. One additional concern is that students and employees may watch these types of training videos online and try to apply the concepts, even if an organization like a school or a corporation does not agree with the approach. This could result in one or more people attacking an armed subject who is not an active shooter and causing a shooting.

Some experts have advocated these approaches for schools since at least 2006, when a contractor was hired by a school system in Burleson, Texas, to train more than 8,000 K–12 students to attack an active shooter. The approach was so controversial that it drew considerable national media attention. Since that time, the debate about this approach has been intense, with many educators firmly opposed to the idea, major insurance carriers deeply skeptical of it, and police heavily divided.

Special operations teams and police tactical personnel routinely use distraction techniques to rescue hostages. Explosive simulators, often referred to as "flash bangs," are used to momentarily distract and disorient armed aggressors to buy precious seconds for tactical personnel to kill or subdue them. Though aggressors have killed some hostages during rescue attempts using this technique, it can also work extremely well, as it did when employed by the Royal Dutch Marines to rescue hostages being held by terrorists in a school in 1977 (Terrorists, 1977).

The use of distraction by the Royal Dutch Marines and many other tactical units proves that this method can buy some time for rescuers to take action. At the same time, there is a considerable difference between what highly trained and experienced tactical personnel can do under life and death stress and what we can reasonably expect from the average civilian who has not practiced extensively. Jacob Ryker was ready, able, and willing to attack an active shooter in spite of having been shot and wounded; however, not everyone has the ability to perform the same way under similar circumstances. A number of attempts by unarmed students and staff to disarm aggressors in schools have not ended so well. Our research determined that at least five people have died trying to disarm armed individuals in American schools to date (Dorn and Satterly, 2012).

Perhaps one of the most challenging aspects is the need for judgment. Law enforcement officers in the state of Georgia complete three full days of training on the judgmental use of deadly force before they are certified. This does not count the hundreds of hours of training they receive on the techniques of safely handling and using a gun, shooting skills, range qualification, or the legal aspects of using a gun in self-defense and more. This training is strictly focused on making the decision to shoot or not to shoot. During this training, officers are exposed to a wide array of scenarios to help them practice how to rapidly recognize the situations they may be faced with on the street. Officers do not practice primarily for active shooters because this would leave them ill prepared to recognize other dangerous situations and react to them quickly.

When Should We Fight?

The student was clearly agitated when he pulled the high-capacity semiautomatic pistol from his pocket and jammed the muzzle into the side of his head. The school principal could see the boy's finger firmly on the gun's trigger, his hand shaking noticeably. He could hear the quivering in the boy's voice as he threatened to kill himself. The students near the boy begged him not to shoot and to put the gun down. The principal knew that he had mere seconds to take action to prevent a tragedy. Without hesitation, he decided that he must attack the gunman.

Fortunately, the high school principal who made this decision did so in a controlled simulation rather than in a real event. Had this been a real situation, the principal would likely be responsible for the death of a student. He would have increased rather than decreased the danger to other students and staff. With this response, he might have needlessly lost his own life as well. By misapplying a concept designed specifically for active shooter situations, the principal's actions would make it more likely that the boy would respond defensively and cause mass casualties.

Luckily, that boy with the gun was only a simulation in a realistic video used to test how educators would respond to a crisis. Since two public school students and one Catholic school student had killed, or attempted to kill, themselves with handguns at school within the months preceding this simulation (Jones, 2013; Student committed, 2013; Ortiz, 2013), the scenario used was not unrealistic. In fact, this situation is actually statistically more likely than an incident like Sandy Hook or Columbine.

Because this was only a simulation, the principal would not be sued, and more importantly, he did not have to live with the consequences of one or more deaths caused by his dangerous reaction. But the principal who made this decision was not at fault. Like the nuns at the Our Lady of Angels Sacred Hearts School and the teacher at the Red Lake Reservation School, the principal had been inadvertently conditioned to fail. The principal had recently watched the video *Run, Hide, Fight*, and, like other educators who have participated in our simulations after viewing this video, his ability to make life and death decisions appeared to have been seriously degraded rather than enhanced by the experience.

But how could this short video possibly cause such a bizarre reaction? While the narrative of the video clearly and repeatedly instructs viewers that they should only attack an active shooter as a last resort, there is no mention in the video of people threatening to kill themselves. There is also no mention of the fact that many people who brandish guns each year do not shoot anyone, or that an attacker might take hostages instead of killing anyone.

To illustrate how this can be an important detail, here is one verbal scenario we use with school staff members:

> You are supervising a group of students outside of your school. You are located about 25 yards from an exterior door to the school and you have a key or access control fob to that door. You notice a man, who appears to be angry, walking towards you and the children. The man is about 75 yards away—this is about three fourths of the length of a football field. The man is staggering and appears to be intoxicated. You realize that the man has a handgun in one hand. There are no other adults or students outside the school. What would you do?

A typical appropriate response would be to

- take the students quickly back into the school,
- make sure the door closes and is secured,
- notify the office and suggest they implement a lockdown and call 911, or
- take the children to a suitable lockdown location and secure them.

Since the shooting at Sandy Hook Elementary School, we have seen numerous school employees respond to this scenario with statements like "I would attack the gunman because it is now my job to die to protect my students." It is impressive that so many school employees are willing to die to protect their students, but it is distressing that, in most of the scenarios that evoked this reaction, doing so would only increase the danger to school officials and students.

We had never encountered one school employee anywhere in the United States who responded this way to our simulations prior to the shooting at Sandy Hook Elementary School; however, since then a number of school employees have responded that they would send students inside so the staff member could attack or confront the "gunman." When posed with this scenario, some school employees would not even send the students inside but instead state that they would attack the man after telling students to lie on the ground. We have also had a number of school staff respond that they would give their keys or access control fob to elementary-aged students, instruct them to go into the school, and state that they would try to talk to the man with the gun.

It is important to note that these types of responses also place the entire school in danger. This is because none of the school employees who have responded this way have told us that they would notify the school office so a lockdown could be implemented and law enforcement officers could be called. We feel these types of well-intentioned—yet ineffective and potentially deadly—responses are the result of a variety of factors, including the media coverage of the Sandy Hook School shooting, the release of the video *Run, Hide, Fight,* and the media coverage of the increasingly popular recent trend of training programs that teach school employees and students to attack an active shooter.

This type of training might be dangerous in other settings as well. In an active shooter drill held by the Hospital Association of Southern California (HASC), participants were given the option of running, hiding, or fighting. The anecdotal evidence from the drill revealed that many of the participants who had chosen to "run" felt the urge to return to the building to look for friends. More importantly, many of the participants who attacked the gunman were not successful (How to, 2013). It is clear that more evaluation of this approach in different settings is needed, but the results of this drill are aligned with the results we have seen in past incidents as well as our scenario evaluations.

Necessary Cautions

Although we wish there was a simple list of actions that could be applied to all attacks, there is yet no such set of steps that would be correct for all seven of the active shooter events we have been asked to assist with, let alone the broader range of active shooter situations that have taken place around the world. We are concerned that trying to boil complex situations down to a short video or training program that explains a complex concept is an unreliable approach at best and a potentially deadly one at worst.

While children have easily learned to "Stop, Drop, and Roll" if their clothing catches fire, fire is far more predictable in contrast to a determined and heavily armed human being, and even the action steps themselves are easier to implement and require a much smaller range of movement and decision making. Like the example of the Heimlich maneuver, "Stop, Drop, and Roll" is incredibly simplistic compared to the demands of responding to an active shooter.

Conclusion

We have interacted with a number of caring, bright, and highly experienced individuals who advocate these innovative yet controversial approaches. At the same time, the aphorism "the road to hell is paved with good intentions" applies to active shooter response as much as any other situation. We feel that these approaches may be carefully scrutinized during litigation in the future. Even though we rarely offer predictions, we feel that it is likely that people will be killed and/or injured when misapplying these concepts based on our field experience and research. The easiest way for this to happen is a person attacking someone who is armed but has no plans to use the weapon.

At the beginning of this book, we described how the heroic actions of the bookkeeper at McNair Learning Academy in DeKalb County, Georgia, saved lives when she talked down a gunman who had entered her school. Had Ms. Tuff attempted to attack the hostage taker, a multiple-victim shooting would almost assuredly have been triggered. We fervently hope this does not come to fruition and desire that the manner in which these approaches are being presented changes before such a tragedy occurs. In the meantime, we wish to generate a serious discussion to address what we feel has sometimes been a rushed reaction to a very serious and valid concern.

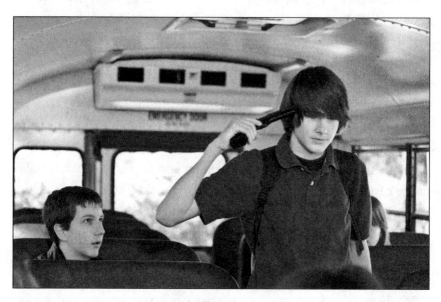

Run, Hide, Fight: Though active shooter training programs emphatically teach that an active shooter should only be attacked as a last resort, many school staff members respond to this video scenario where a student threatens suicide by saying that they would "attack the gunman." As evidenced by past events similar to this scenario, this could be a more dangerous response in many situations. *Photo: Chris Dorn*

This rush to do something about mass casualty shootings has led to many of the problems we have mentioned. This is often true regardless of whether the strategies involve the implementation of security technologies or approaches to improve our response to them once they happen. This trend recurs because of the tremendous emotional impact of tragedies that are intentionally inflicted on innocent people and how much they shock us. This is true no matter how many times similar events occur. Many of the reactions around the nation to the Sandy Hook incident have been even less effective, perhaps because it was such an emotionally charged event due to the location and nature of the attack combined with the tender age of most of the victims.

These tragedies naturally make us all want to do something to make them stop. In each of these cases, people, organizations, and government agencies began implementing dramatic changes before the conclusion of official investigations. This results in actions before we know the actual details of what happened were determined. While we agree that we should be compelled to act instead of waiting on bureaucracy and paperwork, our actions should be guided by reason rather than emotion and a desire to take action for the sole purpose of taking action. While we should debate what can be done and explore new options, it is tragic that we so often ignore concepts that have proven to be effective while we jump to new approaches that may or may not actually work. In other words, we should continue doing what we know works while we consider new alternatives.

Key Points in Chapter Twelve

- At the time of this writing, a variety of theoretical approaches to active shooter response are being implemented that are highly controversial among experts.
- There are indications that some approaches to training people to attack an active shooter may actually increase danger in certain situations.
- The options of running, hiding, or fighting during an active shooter incident can be either an effective or a deadly choice depending on the context.
- It is illogical and dangerous to disregard all other hazards and focus only on active shooter situations.
- Running can slow evacuation times when large numbers of people are in any location with limited exit points.
- People who rush for exits often jam up exit-ways and cause delays that could be truly catastrophic as people pile up in egress routes.

- Moving briskly and with purpose to escape from outdoor danger can reduce the chances that people will be trampled while reducing evacuation time.
- A gunman may have a higher hit rate when victims try to flee from a simulated attacker in a zigzag pattern.
- It can be very difficult to tell where the sound of gunfire is coming from during an attack.

BIBLIOGRAPHY

Controversial city of Houston video: Run, hide, fight. (2012). *KHOU.com*. Retrieved from *http://www.khou.com/news/local/HPD-shooting-164903426.html*.

Cullen, D. (2009). *Columbine*. New York: Twelve.

Dorn, M. (2012). Safe topics: The first 30 seconds. *Safe Topics*. Macon, GA: Safe Havens International.

Dorn, M., and S. Satterly. (2012). Fight, flight or lockdown: Teaching students and staff to attack active shooters could result in decreased casualties or needless deaths. Macon, GA: Safe Havens International.

How to plan an active shooter drill. (2013). Retrieved October 15, 2013, from *http://www.regroup.com/welcome/how-to-plan-an-active-shooter-drill/*

Iroquois Theatre fire. (2007). Retrieved July 8, 2013, from *http://www.eastlandmemorial.org/iroquois.shtml*

Jones, E. (2013). Michigan middle school student commits suicide in school bathroom. *Heavy*. Retrieved from *http://www.heavy.com/news/2013/03/michigan-middle-school-student-commits-suicide-in-school-bathroom/*

Kenya Mall attack survivor played dead to live. (2013). CNN.com, October 10th, 2013. Retrieved from *http://www.cnn.com/2013/10/10/world/africa/kenya-mall-attack-survivor/index.html*

Lifeguarding. (2013). Retrieved July 12, 2013, *from http://www.redcross.org/take-a-class/program-highlights/lifeguarding*

Longman, J. (1998). Shootings in a schoolhouse: The hero; Wounded teenager is called a hero. *The New York Times*. Retrieved from *http://www.nytimes.com/1998/05/23/us/shootings-in-a-schoolhouse-the-hero-wounded-teen-ager-is-called-a-hero.html*

Medina, J. (2009). *Brain rules: 12 principles for surviving and thriving at work, home, and school*. Seattle: Pear Press.

Ola, L. (2013). Gunmen kill 28 in attack on northeast Nigeria school. *Reuters.* Retrieved from *http://www.reuters.com/article/2013/07/06/us-nigeria-violence-idUSBRE96505F20130706*

Ortiz, E. (2013). Ohio high school student 'struggled' with gun before trying to commit suicide in classroom: report. *Daily News.* Retrieved from *http://www.nydailynews.com/news/national/suicidal-ohio-student-struggled-gun-report-article-1.1330979*

Ready Houston (Producer). (2012, July 12, 2013). Run, hide, fight: Surviving an active shooter event. Retrieved from *http://www.youtube.com/watch?v=5VcSwejU2D0*

Ripley, A. (2008). *The unthinkable: Who survives when disaster strikes and why.* New York: Three Rivers Press.

School teacher refused him. (1900, May 13). *The New York Times.* Retrieved from *http://query.nytimes.com/mem/archive-free/pdf?res=F10713FD3F5911738DDD AA0994DD405B808CF1D3*

Student committed suicide at Coweta School. (2013). *FOX23.com.* Retrieved from *http://www.fox23.com/news/local/story/Student-committed-suicide-at-Coweta-school/-jXVNgYkP0GvgEbGzn5Lhg.cspx*

Students taught to attack if gunman appears. (2008). *Education on NBCNews. com.* Retrieved from *http://www.nbcnews.com/id/15253321/ns/us_news-education/t/students-taught-attack-if-gunman-appears/#.UeBIilOvt7Y*

Terrorists: The commandos strike at dawn. (1977). *Time Magazine.* Retrieved from *http://www.time.com/time/magazine/article/0,9171,915035,00.html*

VanMeenen, K. R. S., R. M. DeMarco, F. B. Chua, N. Janal, et al. (2006). Suppression: Sound and light interference with targeting. *Proceedings, 6219.* doi: 10.1117/12.666107.

Yao, L. (2013). Man detained for fatal school stabbing attack. ChinaDaily.com.cn. Retrieved from *http://www.chinadaily.com.cn/china/2013-01/17/content_16128905.htm*

CHAPTER THIRTEEN

HOPE, CONFIDENCE, AND RESILIENCE AS TOOLS FOR SURVIVAL: YOU CAN DO THIS!

Confidence and adaptability can help you survive deadly encounters and thrive in their aftermath.

On the night of June 27, 2005, a four-man SEAL team fast roped out of a helicopter into a remote part of Afghanistan on a mission named Operation Red Wings. The four members of the SEAL reconnaissance and surveillance team were Team Leader Navy Lieutenant Michael Murphy, Petty Officer Second Class Danny Dietz, Petty Officer Second Class Matthew Axelson, and SO-1 Marcus Luttrell (Luttrell, 2007). The goal of this mission was the development of intelligence on a Taliban commander.

The team moved to their position overlooking their target area and began their surveillance. Shortly thereafter, some Afghani goat herders accidently discovered the soldiers and were taken prisoner by the SEALs. Determining that they were civilians, Lieutenant Murphy ordered their release, as required by their Rules of Engagement and the Geneva Conventions. This turned out to be a critical decision point for the four men when a sizable force of Taliban *mujahidin*, presumably warned by the released goat herders, attacked the team.

During the attack, which came from three directions, the SEALs were subjected to fire from rifles, machine guns, rocket-propelled grenades, and mortar rounds. The SEALs were forced to abandon their position several times in order to prevent themselves from being overrun. Lieutenant Murphy was fatally wounded after moving out of cover into an open field to get reception for their satellite radio in an attempt to call for help. The call briefly got through to their headquarters. Eventually, Murphy, Axelson, and Dietz were killed during the gun battle.

At one point during the fight, a rocket-propelled grenade exploded near Luttrell and Axelson, flinging them both away from their position. Luttrell was rendered unconscious. When he regained consciousness, Taliban fighters were looking for him, and though severely injured, he began to evade them. During his evasion, he fell short distances down the mountainside. In one of his many slides down the steep slopes, he ended up suspended upside down and was subsequently shot in his left thigh. Luttrell sustained numerous scrapes and bruises and fractured three of his vertebrae. He had also received numerous shrapnel wounds during the attack and was losing blood at a steady rate (Luttrell, 2007).

Despite his injuries, he crawled away and evaded capture by the Taliban forces for six days. He walked four miles and crawled three more before he met a group of friendly Pashtun villagers. Thankfully, the Pashtun village leader invoked an ancient Pashtun concept they call *lokhay warkawal*, or tribal hospitality. Due to the friendship of this village, his wounds were treated, and he was protected from the Taliban, even after the Taliban threatened to destroy the village for sheltering an American. For his role in the attack and the subsequent heroism in escape and evasion while injured, SO-1 Marcus Luttrell was awarded the Navy Cross, the second highest award for bravery in the U.S. military.

Prior to his enlistment in the Navy, Lutrell was trained by Reno Alberto. Alberto is a former SEAL who trains young men both mentally and physically for the rigors of Basic Underwater Demolition School. Reno once told him, "It's the mind that needs training." Throughout his Afghani ordeal, Luttrell had cause to remember those words (Luttrell, 2007).

This story, which was being made into a film starring Mark Wahlberg at the time of this writing, is an excellent example of how we sometimes can complete extraordinary tasks when all odds are against us. In this chapter, we will discuss how powerful our mind can be, if it is trained, in helping us effectively respond to a crisis.

How to Improve Your Crisis Resilience

Nobody *wants* to fail in a crisis, but some of us prepare to do so inadvertently. There are those of us who take steps to prepare, and then there are those who fail to prepare, and thus are preparing to fail. Abe's preparation by taking training in martial arts saved his life and the lives of four others. Marcus Luttrell's training saved his life in Afghanistan. How can you take advantage of these same techniques without knowing what threat you might face?

We have introduced you to numerous skills like threat assessment, ways to build situational awareness, pattern matching and recognition to detect danger, and mental simulation to allow for stress inoculation. None of these skills will help you at all if you do not train yourself to use them, and use them well. One of the goals of training is to develop muscle memory. When a crisis occurs and your heart rate rises, you lose cognitive function and some manual dexterity. If you have developed muscle memory, your body will perform without thinking.

Reloading a gun in the middle of a shootout is a prime example of a skill that needs to be trained into muscle memory. Though a relatively simple action with a semiautomatic pistol, it can still be extremely challenging to reload while being shot at. The simple steps of pressing a button to drop an empty magazine, grabbing a loaded magazine, properly orienting it to the gun, pushing it into the magazine well, slapping it on the bottom to make sure it is seated properly, releasing the slide of the weapon to chamber the first round of ammunition, and firing the weapon takes considerable practice. To be able to perform these steps in a gunfight at 3:00 A.M. requires even more extensive hands-on experience. Practicing and training can dramatically help improve your ability to respond to crisis situations and save lives.

One man who can attest to this is Tom Satterly. Tom recently retired from the U.S. Army after serving 25 years, most of them in Special

Operations. His first four years were spent as a combat engineer in the 54th Engineer Battalion in Wildflecken, Germany. When Tom reenlisted, he went through Special Forces Qualifications, passed, and joined the 5th Special Forces Group, stationed in Ft. Campbell, Kentucky. The life of an elite Green Beret did not satisfy him, so he applied for even more elite schools, specifically the Selection Course for the Operator Training Course (OTC)—the training for what we know as the "Delta Force."

In 1991 he made it through Selections and the grueling OTC to become a Delta Operator just as the First Gulf War was ending. His first service as an Operator was in Mogadishu, Somalia, where he spent a hellish night of combat in the action that become immortalized in the movie *Blackhawk Down*. For his valorous service in that operation, he was awarded a Bronze Star with a special commendation for valor. During the rest of his military service as an operator, he was involved in missions in Bosnia, Kuwait, Colombia, and Iraq, where he was the leader of the second troop on the scene when Saddam Hussein was captured.

At this time, Special Operations Command (SOCOM) decided to form a new squadron. Tom became one of the first members of this new squadron, which was meant to keep operators constantly deployed rather than having voids of inactivity. He also served in Algeria, Pakistan, and Afghanistan, where he saw combat numerous times. At the end of his service, he had earned five more Bronze Stars, two with special commendations for valor, and he now suffers quietly with his pain from his injuries and the loss of friends in combat.

When Tom was asked how he stayed alive through all these harrowing missions, he simply replied, "Training. Always train" (T. Satterly, personal communication, July 12, 2013). Erwin Rommel, the famous "Desert Fox" from World War II, would agree. He is quoted as saying, "The more you sweat in training; the less you bleed in battle" (Grossman and Christensen, 2011). Proper training has a twofold purpose: to teach the trainee a practical skill and to inoculate the trainee from the stresses he will feel while using that skill under duress.

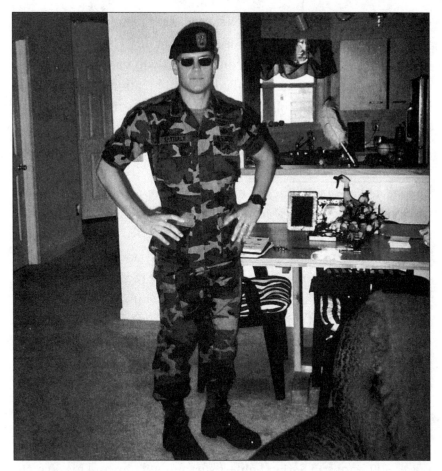

Tom Satterly: Tom Satterly was in combat for 18 straight hours in Mogadishu when he served as a Delta Force Special Operator. Tom was awarded six Bronze Stars before he retired from the Army.
Photo: personal collection of Steve Satterly

Like public safety officials, you should decide what you need to practice, how you will simulate it, and then practice that way, over and over and over. For example, police officers could improve their own training by adding stress to their shooting drills by trying to reload while being timed and having someone fire a pistol nearby to simulate the sounds of a gunfight. They might also simulate the stress of combat by running a few sprints and attempting to change their magazine while their heart rate is elevated. As with any type of drill, adequate safety precautions should be implemented, especially when firearms are involved, loaded or not.

One simple but important concept that you can use when you practice for an emergency is called tactical breathing, or controlled breathing. To use controlled breathing, take in a full breath through your nose while silently counting to four, letting your belly expand, then hold for a count of four before exhaling through your mouth for a count of four, letting your belly deflate. This process should be repeated as many times as necessary as appropriate to slow your heart rate enough to be able to perform the task at hand (Grossman and Christensen, 2011).

The key is to practice each action and slowly add additional skills, committing each to muscle memory. As you practice, take this time to engage in mental simulation. Envision yourself in a situation where you need that skill you are practicing. Visualize yourself being successful. Tom Satterly's advice is, "Never visualize yourself losing" (T. Satterly, personal communication, July 12, 2013). This means that even if you make a mistake, you should visualize yourself correcting it and successfully completing the scenario. If you wonder if this type of training really works, you could ask Captain Zan Hornbuckle, an Army officer during the invasion phase of the war in Iraq. At one point, 300 Iraqi and Syrian fighters surrounded him and his 80 men. Captain Hornbuckle and his unit engaged the enemy for eight hours. In the end, 200 of the enemy were dead, with zero American casualties (Grossman and Christensen, 2011). This success is even more amazing considering that none of Hornbuckle's soldiers had ever been in combat before.

Even though we have used examples from military combat to help convince you of the power of these concepts, you should consider how practicing these simple yet important skills and habits can save your life in everyday situations. For example, you should mentally prepare yourself and practice the important habit of leaving behind your belongings before moving to safety in a crisis. You may need to take your cell phone or radio before retreating to safety so you can call for help, but you should not fall prey to the common tendency for people to take precious time to gather personal items before moving to safety. There are a number of real-life examples of this gathering behavior, including many occupants of the World Trade Center towers who took the time to gather purses, books, and other mundane personal items before evacuating. (Ripley, 2009).

Believing in Yourself

The physical skills needed to survive are absolutely important, but they would be improved tremendously with the belief that you can do what needs to be done. Captain Hornbuckle spent considerable time reminding his men that they could do extraordinary things in battles. He also emphasized that they needed to remember their training. Once the bullets started to fly, one of his primary jobs was to keep his men calm so they could remember their training. Tom Satterly recounts his combat experiences, "If you have to think about what you are going to do, you're lost. I developed confidence in myself because of the training. Don't train to lose. You're never calm, but you are methodical" (T. Satterly, personal communication, July 12, 2013).

There will be times when you get frustrated, mad, and even upset. You may feel sore or get blisters and wonder if the training is worth it. This is natural. But in a life and death situation, you cannot quit. As one SEAL instructor told Luttrell during Basic Underwater Demolition (BUDs) training, "The way out of that is mental—in your mind. Don't buckle under to the hurt; rev up your spirit and your motivation," (Luttrell, 2007). Tom Satterly echoes that sentiment, "Don't give up in your mind. If you do, your body will follow."

One of the main points of SEAL training, Operator training, or Ranger training is to instill in the men who go through that training the belief that they can do whatever has to be done. During the American conflict in Vietnam, two Ranger School graduates found themselves under fire in a rice paddy. Facing a heavy onslaught from the enemy, one looked at the other and said, "Well, hell, at least we're not in Ranger school." (Grossman and Christensen, 2011). You do not need to go through their level of brutal training to feel that same confidence within yourself. Basic personal preparation can help you develop the confidence you need to survive deadly encounters.

But belief in yourself is sometimes not enough. In a crisis, you will rarely ever be responding by yourself, but with others. Even though our favorite movies and TV shows focus on main characters that are "lone wolves," in reality, responding to an emergency is a collaborative effort. Thus, it is important for you to believe in yourself, but it is no less important to believe in others who can help you during a crisis.

When Tom Satterly was in Mogadishu, things were bleak. His unit was in a firefight for 18 hours straight, and it seemed as if they were fighting the entire city. When asked how he got through it, he replied, "I remember thinking, 'Are we ever going to get out of here?' The higher ups, not on the ground, kept covering us with the Little Birds (gunship helicopters), getting the armor together from the Pakistanis. We knew we hadn't been forgotten. You knew the other guys were doing their stuff, so you kept doing what you had to." His belief that others were doing their job was one of the main factors that kept him doing his job.

The Power of the Mind

In 2011, Dave Grossman was interviewed for *The First Thirty Seconds* DVD training and evaluation series. In it he is quoted as saying, "The greatest survival tool the world has ever seen is the properly prepared human brain" (Dorn, 2012). We believe Grossman is correct in this regard. The power of visualization, confidence, and hope are all derived from the human mind.

As Klein points out, there is considerable evidence that our brain can help us make correct life and death decisions with amazing speed and accuracy (Klein, 1998). Tom Satterly and Marcus Luttrell are two prime examples of just how much a human being can do to survive against seemingly impossible odds. While very few people will ever face situations as dire as these men, their drive to survive at all costs affords us powerful lessons that we can all apply. It would be a shame not to learn from their amazing efforts.

Know That You Can Do This!

As you read earlier, stay in touch with yourself, remember your preparation, and visualize yourself successfully completing the task. Above all, maintain hope. Hope is the understanding that, as bad as things might be right now, they will be better. Hope is not a strategy; it is a mindset. Tom Satterly was mired in seemingly endless combat in Mogadishu but never lost hope because he had confidence in his own abilities as well as those on his team.

In a sense, hope is about stubbornness and perseverance. If you know you are doing the right thing, keep doing it. Even if it looks pointless, keep doing it. You may be tired, sore, injured, or scared, but do not quit. Winston Churchill said it best in a speech to Harrow School in 1941, "This is the lesson: never give in, never give in, never, never, never, never—in nothing, great or small, large or petty—never give in except to convictions of honor and good sense. Never yield to force; never yield to the apparently overwhelming might of the enemy" (Churchill, 2013).

When Abe stood up to defend four people against the attacker, all he knew was that he did not want his wife to be hurt. She was first and foremost in his mind as he took on the enraged man armed with a hatchet and a hammer. He did not know if he would survive or not, but he hoped that Erin would. That hope drove his efforts, and he was successful. If you face a deadly situation, and you have hope and belief in yourself, you are more likely to survive even if survival seems but a remote possibility.

Key Points in Chapter Thirteen

- If you have developed muscle memory, your body will more likely perform without thinking.
- Practice mental simulation and visualize yourself being successful.

- Basic personal preparation can help you develop the confidence you need to survive deadly encounters.
- Shock and denial are common stress responses to traumatic events and disasters.
- The urge to do something is your mind's way of taking control of the situation.
- It is important to remember the need to emphasize various positive ways to cope with stress.

BIBLIOGRAPHY

Grossman D., and L. W. Christensen. (2011). *On combat: The psychology and physiology of deadly conflict in war and peace.* Milstadt, IL: Warrior Science Publications.

Dorn, M. (2012). Safe topics: The first 30 seconds. *Safe Topics.* Macon, GA: Safe Havens International.

Klein, G. (1998). *Sources of power: How people make decisions.* Cambridge, MA: The MIT Press.

Luttrell, M. (2007). *Lone survivor: The eyewitness account of Operation. Redwing and the lost heroes of SEAL Team 10.* New York: Hachette Digital.

Ripley, A. (2008). *The Unthinkable: Who Survives When Disaster Strikes—and Why.* New York: Three Rivers Press.

Winston Churchill: Famous quotations and speeches. (2013). Retrieved July 7, 2013, from *http://www.winstonchurchill.org/learn/speeches/quotations*

CHAPTER FOURTEEN

STRESS AND TRAUMATIC STRESS

How you see it is how it will be.

It was a beautiful day in Nigeria, as beautiful as any other. Akintayo smiled as he left his home and walked to where his friend lived. He walked along, daydreaming just like any other boy his age. The day was beautiful, the world seemed alive, and the possibilities were endless.

When Akintayo got to his friend's house, he and some other kids sat on the front porch for a bit to discuss their plans for the day. They decided to play some soccer, so they entered the house to get some food to take with them. The boy greeted his friend's parents, and he watched as his friend's mother gathered some fried meats and fruits in a bag. She added a canteen of water, and his friend came in with a soccer ball.

The mother looked up and out of the window and let out a gasp. With urgency, she turned to the boys and said, "Quickly! Out the back!"

Before the boys could even register what she had said, the front door burst open and several men with guns stormed inside. One of the first men in the door shot into the ceiling, sending everyone into a state of shock and freezing them into immobility.

The man who had fired into the ceiling began yelling, "You! Get into that room!" He pointed, and the other men with guns herded everyone into the room yelling and pushing to get compliance.

In the room, they forced everyone down on the floor. The adults began crying out, knowing what was to come, and then the youngest began to cry. Akintayo wanted to defend himself, but he couldn't seem to make his body move. It got worse when the shots rang out as they executed the people on the floor.

Akintayo's immobility most likely saved his life. He was shot in the shoulder, and his lack of movement must have convinced the killers that he was dead. He survived the terrible event, but despite the gunshot wound to his shoulder, the loss of his friends, and the tremendous stress of the event, Akintayo Kolawole Akinlade considers himself lucky to be alive. Rather than let this event define his life, Akintayo developed a positive outlook on life that he has passed on to his family.

"That experience makes me thankful to be alive today, and I don't take my days here on earth for granted." He smiles as he recounts what can only be described as a horrendous experience: "I was scared and praying to be able to see my family again. They locked us in a room and I remember people screaming but I could not move. I thought I was going to die." (A. Akinlade, personal communication, 2013).

As he recounted the event, he pointed to the bullet wound on his shoulder, wiped a tear from his eye, and said, "No young child should go through that. I'm grateful to be alive and that I got to grow up. Some of my friends that day never got that chance." Akintayo is now an American citizen, the proud and caring father of two children and a kind husband.

The *Oxford Dictionary* defines stress as "pressure or tension exerted on a material object." Pressure on our brains and/or tension on our bodies can cause a great deal of stress. Pressure can come from a variety of things, ranging from work to family to our daily environment. Understanding stress is an age-old quest. Hundreds of studies are devoted to the subject, yet we have not quite figured out the magic solution to controlling stress. Perhaps it is because stress cannot be avoided. No matter what we do on this earth, there is a certain amount of stress involved. This stress is both good and bad for us. However, our focus should not be directly aimed at avoiding stress. Instead, a focus on reducing the negative stress and harnessing the overwhelming pangs of emotional discourse can create a tapestry of emotional release. In other words, we can sometimes turn the bad things that worry us into something positive.

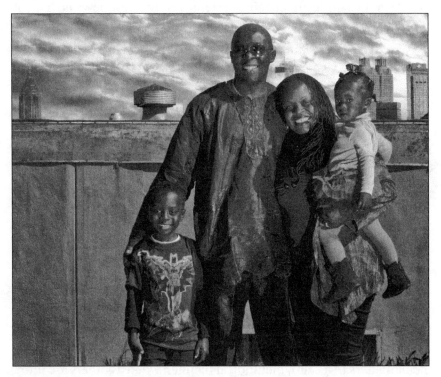

Akintayo: Having survived a horrific attack as a teen, Akintayo Akinlade makes it a point to live life to the fullest and bring joy to his family each day.
Photo: Rachel Wilson

Rising above an emotional tidal wave is a stressful thought in and of itself. But survival is human nature. Surviving stressful situations is what we are built for. Imagine that you are in an empty parking garage. As you begin to walk to your car, you hear footsteps in the distance. You turn your head in the direction of the sound. Your heart begins to beat faster, and your entire body is ready to respond. In this scenario, would you not want your brain to react to the stress of the situation? Thanks to evolution, it will. Your brain will sound a clarion call to the rest of your body, which will tell your heart to beat faster, thus increasing your blood pressure, in turn causing you to breathe faster. This has the end result of making your heart and lungs pump more oxygenated blood to your muscles. Your liver will then release more sugar into your blood stream and get you ready to perform. It is quite an amazing system, and the best news is that you are already a proud owner of this advanced technology!

We have evolved into a species poised and ready to handle a great deal of stress. We are equipped with a highly skilled brain and an adaptive drive, so we already have what it takes to survive. As you have seen already, you can also learn to activate some aspects of this highly developed survival mode consciously. But if an automatic unconscious switch controls this survival mode, how can we learn to turn it on and off with a higher degree of control?

In order to tap into these stress survival skills, it is important to understand that not everyone will handle stress equally. Some stress-ors clearly can be traced to individual factors (e.g., personality, social support, coping skills), whereas others are environmental factors (e.g., work, family life, financial situations). For the most part, people vary widely in terms of how much stress they can withstand, how much they let it get to them, and how much they may transmit it to those around them. Some people are emotionally predisposed to handle dif-ficult matters in a calm, methodical manner, whereas others are prone to lose control and "freak out" when faced with difficult situations.

Do not despair if you are one of those personality types that is not as comfortable with high-stress situations. According to researcher Joel Paris, environmental factors are a great determinant in your mental health status, whether you are predisposed to adequately handle stress or not (Paris, 1999). In other words, even the person with a weak stress constitution can perform amazing feats if the envi-ronment is right for that person. You have probably heard stories of courageous behavior in times of crisis. For example, people can learn to lead a happy and fulfilling life after experiencing even the worst of life's most violent encounters.

As a case in point, most folks in North Georgia and Tennessee knew Raleigh Cooper as "Bud." Bud was one of those modest, quiet, kind, generous men who focused on making those around him happy while also enjoying life himself. Bud revered his wife and adored his children. He was equally revered and loved by them. He served as a Boy Scout leader and as a Deacon in his church. He would also stop on the side of the road to help anyone who was broken down, even when most people might not think it was safe to do so. Bud Cooper was all of these things, no matter how much tragedy he experienced.

One day, while enjoying one of his favorite pastimes—fishing— he snagged something heavy with his lure. When he reeled in the object, he was shocked to see that it was a boy who had drowned. This terrible experience haunted Bud for some time. But life had more challenges for Bud Cooper. Shortly after retiring from his job driving a delivery truck, he badly cut his arm while cutting firewood with a chain saw in the woods. He was barely able to make it to the road where a pulpwood truck driver found him and rushed him to the hospital. If he had not made it to the hospital so quickly he would have died from his injury. Of course, Bud kept on going strong in life.

But Bud had another life experience that made these other stories pale in comparison. As a young pharmacist's mate in the Navy, Bud was one of thousands of Americans who landed on the beaches at Normandy in June of 1944. He was spared the grisly first day of the landing because his ship had hit a mine and was delayed in reaching the shore. When he arrived the day after the initial landing, one of his duties was tending to the wounded and helping to retrieve the thousands of bodies scattered up and down the beach, bloated from sitting out in the sun for a full day. His time on the beach was cut short when he was hit by a German machine gun round that ripped through his torso.

After recovering in a British hospital, he went on to serve in the push across Europe, and he later served briefly in the South Pacific before the end of the war. But of all the places and things that he saw during his service, nothing could compare to the scene he saw on the beach that day in Normandy. He once said there was no way to convey the horrors of that fateful beach to someone who did not see it firsthand. Years later, he would find it nearly impossible to describe to anyone what he witnessed in that Hell on earth. Regardless of how incredible special effects technology has become, he maintained that no movie could truly begin to capture the horror, nor replicate the terrible sounds, smells, and grisly sights of D-Day.

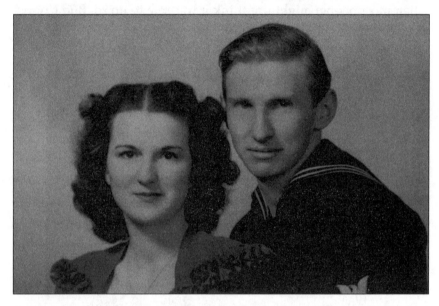

Bud Cooper: Bud Cooper saw the horrors of the beach landing at Normandy and survived a gunshot wound to serve again in the Pacific Theater. Bud led a full, happy, and productive life after the war, bringing much joy to his family and friends. *Photo: personal collection of the Cooper family*

A world away from Chattanooga, Tennessee, in a dramatically different culture, Tao Nguyen also witnessed extreme tragedy. His wife and four daughters all died during the prolonged conflict that the Vietnamese now refer to as "the American War." One of his daughters died from illness and another was accidently shot by a Vietnamese soldier who was flirting with her. Later, his wife and remaining two children were killed in a car accident. Somehow, Tao remarried and raised a stepdaughter, a son and two more daughters. Mr. Nguyen died of cancer in 1994 after spending many joyful years with his beloved children—children who also loved him dearly. Somehow, like Bud Cooper, Mr. Nguyen found a way to find joy after experiencing tragedy that is beyond the ability of most people to comprehend. Bud Cooper, like millions of soldiers from hundreds of terrible wars around the globe, found solace in his fishing and hunting trips, frequent worship, and the countless hours he spent making his family happy. Like many parents who have experienced the deep pain of losing a family, Tao Nguyen found a way not only to carry on with his life but also to make the lives of those around him blossom and thrive.

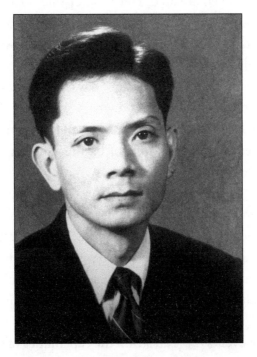

Tao Nguyen: Tao Nguyen lost his wife and four daughters to war, but was able to recover and start a new family to continue his life journey.
Photo: personal collection of the Nguyen family

Disaster can also come from mass casualty incidents caused by severe weather and other natural disasters. In recognition of those who have faced this kind of personal challenge, Oprah Winfrey acknowledged several unsung heroes who rose to the occasion during Hurricane Katrina. Makeba, a pharmacist at a hospital in

New Orleans, was one of them. She reported to work as the ferocious storm headed her way. The hospital administrators told Makeba she could go home, but she knew patients needed medication, even with a category five hurricane rolling in.

While the storm raged outside, Makeba worked around the clock. After three days with no sleep, Makeba reached her breaking point and the stress of the situation began to sink in. She began thinking about her home and the beloved pets she had left behind. She called her mother and told her she was leaving the hospital. "I was crying my heart out," Makeba related. Her mother said, "You have patients that are depending on you. When you graduated from school, you took an oath to serve, and if you walk out, you're walking out on everything that you stand for." Makeba's mother's words gave her the strength to stay on duty for 10 straight days, filling prescriptions and delivering life-saving medications to people in need (Winfrey, 2005). Makeba was able to rise above the pressure of the storm and continue to work. The emotional reactions of crying, thinking about family members, and reaching out to others are natural survival responses when humans are faced with stress.

Our mind and body will do whatever it takes to cope with extreme stress. It is important to listen to your body and take care of yourself. Crisis stress can also garner its own types of issues inherent to the situation. For example, shootings with a high death toll are classified as mass casualty events and present their own unique stress challenges. Although infrequent, mass casualty incidents are potentially overwhelming events that can strain the capabilities of even the most organized emergency medical services, hospitals, public safety agencies, communities, and, often, the nation.

The Boston Marathon bombing incident and the school-shooting incident at Sandy Hook Elementary School shook our nation to its core. In each case, we watched a mass casualty incident unfold before our very eyes. In one instance, we were shocked by the age of the victims as well as how brutally their lives were taken from us. The type of stress we felt as a country was multiplied exponentially, and most of us felt some sort of response on a personal level. In each instance, the nation stood in shock, horror, and rage as we learned of innocent lives being lost. These people were just like many of us, and those children feel just like our own. We wept together during memorials for the victims, and we are healing together as we try to make sense of what happened.

Some stresses are extraordinary and thus require extraordinary attention to resolve them. We refer to them as "traumatic stress." This type of stress is defined as the reaction to any challenge, demand, threat, or change that exceeds our coping resources and results in distress (Headington Institute, 2011). There are certain symptoms and reactions to traumatic stress that must be noted. Typically, shock and denial are common stress responses to traumatic events and disasters, especially shortly after the event. Both shock and denial are normal, protective reactions. Shock is a sudden and often intense disturbance of your emotional state that may leave you feeling stunned or dazed. Denial keeps us from acknowledging that something very stressful has happened, or from fully experiencing the intensity of the event. You may temporarily feel numb or disconnected from life. Again, these are normal reactions to abnormal events.

Some people will experience traumatic stress reactions from watching tragic events on television; others will fantasize about what they would do if they were faced with a similar situation; others will volunteer, make donations, or participate in some other type of activity to assuage the mental anguish they are feeling. Many will talk about it at work, school, at a social gathering, or at home. All of these things are normal stress reactions. The urge to do something is your mind's way of taking control of the situation.

To assist in your mind's effort to take action, it is important for everyone, including families, schools, workplaces, and faith-based organizations to make a plan for how to help yourself and others during any type of stressful incident—particularly mass casualty incidents. Doing so will actually help you alleviate stress while preparing you for the next crisis. According to the *Jane's Citizen Safety*

Guide, it is recommended that your plans cover at least seventy-two hours of interrupted services (Shepherd et al, 2004). Think about it this way: what would you do if you and your family were faced with an event so large that help—including police, fire, emergency medical, and other 911 services—could not get to you for 72 hours? How would you survive? Write down your plan and make sure your family and loved ones know the plan. Grossman points out that this type of planning can not only help us improve our ability to respond to a crisis, but can help us to recover more effectively as well (Grossman and Christensen, 2011).

According the American Psychological Association, as the initial shock subsides, stress reactions (including traumatic stress reactions) vary from one person to another. It is important to note that there is no wrong or right way to feel. The tips and lists mentioned in this chapter are intended to provide you with information about traumatic stress in general; they are not meant to serve as an indication or diagnosis of any particular disorders. The following, however, are normal responses to a traumatic event (Managing traumatic stress, 2011):

- **Intense and unpredictable feelings that may seem overwhelming.** You may become more annoyed than usual, and your mood may fluctuate dramatically. You might be especially anxious or nervous, or even depressed and angry.
- **Thoughts and behavior patterns are affected by the trauma.** You might have repeated and vivid memories of the event. These flashbacks may occur for no apparent reason and may lead to physical reactions such as rapid heartbeat or sweating. You may find it difficult to concentrate or make decisions, or you may become more easily confused. Sleep and eating patterns also may be disrupted. You may also experience an intense startle reflex, which means you will startle very easily, and hypersensitivity to anything that surprises you, like unexpected loud noises.
- **Triggers may prompt reactions even after the event has passed.** Anniversaries of the event can trigger upsetting memo-

ries of the traumatic experience. These "triggers" may be accompanied by fears that the stressful event will be repeated.

- **Relationships may be impacted.** Greater conflict, such as more frequent arguments with family members and coworkers, is common. On the other hand, you might become withdrawn and isolated and avoid your usual activities.

- **You may experience physical reactions.** For example, headaches, nausea, and chest pain may result and may require medical attention. Preexisting medical conditions may worsen with increased stress as well.

Other traumatic stress reactions can be categorized as Psychological, Cognitive, Behavioral, Physical, and Spiritual (Boan, 2012). More specifically, the Humanitarian Disaster Relief Institute outlines specific reactions within each category in their publication *Disaster Spiritual and Emotional Care Tip Sheets*. These tips indicate that people who experience severe trauma can have several common reactions including anger, sadness, memory problems, confusion, changes in activity levels, muscle soreness, menstrual cycle changes, and questioning of one's faith. Anyone can experience these types of symptoms. You do not have to actually be in a crisis event to have traumatic stress reactions. For example, here is how a Humanitarian Disaster Relief Worker recounts her experience as she was preparing to respond to the conflict in Kosovo:

> The period before deployment was extremely stressful. There was so much to do and my experience made me feel inadequately prepared. My immediate medical chain of command seemed to offer little or no support or advice. In Kosovo I spent seven extremely demanding months. I felt completely responsible for ensuring that nothing would go wrong. I knew that I was pushing myself too hard and neglecting my own personal needs, but I wasn't able to let up. (Weine et al., 2002)

If you experience or know of anyone who experiences any of these symptoms, there are coping mechanisms to counteract these overwhelming feelings. It is possible, and even highly probable, that you will get through the stressful times that accompany a disaster. Whether helping yourself, an individual, or even several dozen people in the wake of a mass casualty event, it is important to remember the need to emphasize various positive ways to cope with stress. We will further explore coping mechanisms in the next chapter.

The common view of stress being a minor factor in our lives is not accurate. It is commonplace for people to view stress as a little problem here or a small issue there. Research has shown that stress can have an array of harmful effects on your mind and body. It can fuel cancer and contribute to heart attacks. In some instances, it can be the source of depression and anxiety.

Conclusion

The survivor mentality is important to recovering from any crisis. We are all survivors, and this is evidenced by the fact that our species has endured and evolved for millions of years. Though Akintayo Akinlade, Bud Cooper, and Tao Nguyen never had the benefit of the vast research that has been conducted in the decades since they each found themselves faced with immeasurable pain, they were able to find some way to move forward in spite of what they experienced. Their success stories, and the others we have shared throughout this book, demonstrate how resilient people can be at coping with even massive amounts of stress no matter what society we live in, what age we are, or what worldview we hold.

If you look around you, you can find survivors just like these three men almost anywhere. The authors know this because these outstanding men are all members of our families. More importantly, these are just a few typical examples of the people in our lives and yours that hold these qualities. Just as we encountered them, you have or will surely encounter others who have also risen to the challenges life can throw at anyone, anywhere in the world. There have been millions of others who have also been able to find a way to carry on in a meaningful way, to bring much joy to those they interact with in life. The children, grandchildren, and other descendants of these ordinary yet amazing men prove their achievements were well worthwhile.

Make no mistake about it; you are here because someone in your lineage survived a crisis situation. With the information that is now available to us, we know this resiliency can be enhanced if we apply these concepts along with the age-old power of the human being to persevere. Efforts to continue to bring joy to a world that is always in need of rays of hope sometimes give the greatest meaning to life. Learn to be a survivor, not just for yourself, but for all those whose destinies you shape.

Key Points in Chapter Fourteen

- Survival is human nature. Surviving stressful situations is what we are built for.
- Our mind and body will do whatever it takes to cope with extreme stress.
- There are a variety of physical and mental reactions to traumatic crisis situations. Proper mental preparation can protect against some of these negative reactions, but in some cases these natural responses can save our lives.

BIBLIOGRAPHY

Boan, J. A. D. (2012). *Tip Sheet: Recognizing common survivor stress reactions.* Wheaton, IL: Wheaton College Humanitarian Disaster Institute.

Grossman, D., and L. W. Christensen. (2011). On combat: The psychology and physiology of deadly conflict in war and peace. Milstadt, IL: Warrior Science Publications.

Headington Institute: Care of Caregivers Worldwide. (2011). Retrieved May 31, 2013, from *http://www.headington-institute.org/*

Managing traumatic stress: Tips for recovering from disasters and other traumatic events. (2011, August). Retrieved May 31, 2013, from *http://www.apa.org/helpcenter/recovering-disasters.aspx*

Paris, J. (1999). *Nature and nuture in psychiatry: A predisposition-stress model of mental disorders.* Washington, DC: American Psychiatric Press.

Shepherd, S., J. B. C., R. M. Fanney, R. Campbell, A. Dwyer, and J. Duda. (2004). *Jane's Citizen's Safety Guide.* Surrey, United Kingdom: Jane's Information Group.

Weine, S. D. Y., D. Silove, M. Van Ommeren, J. A. Fairbank, and J. Saul. (2002). Guidelines for international training in mental health and psychosocial interventions for trauma exposed populations in clinical and community settings. *Psychiatry, 65*(2), 156–164.

Winfrey, O. (2005, November 21). True American Heroes. *Oprah's favorite things 2005.* Retrieved May 27, 2013, from *http://www.oprah.com/oprahshow/True-American-Heroes/1#ixzz2UQelD5rB*

CHAPTER FIFTEEN

HOW TO COPE EFFECTIVELY

It may not be easy but you can recover from tragedy.

Mrs. Abi was the mother of 18 children. Not only was she the matriarch of the family, but she was also grandmother, cook, maid, and babysitter. She was beloved by her children, and they were all a tight-knit unit.

One country morning on their family farm, Mrs. Abi was babysitting her six-year-old granddaughter as she did every weekend. It was just an average morning, but this particular day would change her life forever. As her granddaughter played in their modest house, Mrs. Abi hung her clothes outside to dry. Suddenly she heard a frightful scream coming from her kitchen. As she ran into the house, she noticed flames. She soon saw her granddaughter engulfed in a fiery blaze. Horrified and frightened, she jumped on her granddaughter, using her body to put out the fire. But it was too late. The child lay lifeless on the ground, and Mrs. Abi had severe burns and charred skin. She was so distraught she did not even notice her severe burns at the time.

The tragedy broke the family bond she had with her children. She was wracked by guilt, and she and her daughter had an equally hard time coping with the loss of a beloved child. After years of counseling and what seemed like an ocean of tears, they learned to get through the difficult times.

Fifty years later, Mrs. Abi still bears the memory of that dreadful day, and she still has the scars from it. She decided against surgery and skin grafts to clear her physical wounds. She felt that the wounds would heal along with her heart—without help, without medicine. She needed to see herself heal physically and, somehow in her mind, seeing her burnt skin reminded her of her granddaughter's precious life.

Her daughter had to not only cope with the loss of her child but she also had to learn to forgive and love her mother again. The process took several years, but their family grew even closer. She took care of her aging mother for more than 20 years after her father died, and held her mother's hand when she died.

Mrs. Abi and her daughter were able to go through the hard time after the disaster with the help of professional counseling and family support. This chapter will examine different means of coping that can help you get through tragedy should you ever have to face it.

Negative Coping Mechanisms

The silver lining to the stress cloud is the fact that there are hundreds of coping strategies. At the same time, not all strategies are positive. According to the authors of the popular book *Wellness: Concepts and Applications*, negative coping mechanisms include violence, overeating, not eating, consuming alcoholic beverages, consuming large amounts of caffeine, smoking, and using drugs (Anspaugh, 2006). These types of behaviors are referred to as negative coping strategies because of their negative impacts on the mind, body, and soul. The Department of Veteran Affairs—National Center for Post Traumatic Stress Disorder (PTSD) recommends that you avoid using negative coping mechanisms as they may severely hamper your ability to cope and interfere with healthy healing.

Avoidance

Sometimes places, people, and even smells may remind you of the trauma. At first it seems natural to avoid these triggers, but the opposite may be true. The goal of crisis stabilization is to be able to integrate the traumatic event into your life without experiencing the overwhelming feelings. In order to achieve this goal, you will need social supports—supports from family, friends, the community. But when you avoid going out to places and meeting with people, it will not only tune out supports for you but also make you feel even more isolated and bring on negative thoughts. Even when you feel like being alone, it is crucial that you try to get out and rejoin society. More than ever, this is the time that you need to participate in social activities and rally around loved ones.

Extraordinarily Heightened Sense of Alert

After going through a trauma, you may think that it is logical to stay extremely vigilant, always looking out for danger. For a soldier on patrol in a combat zone this might be appropriate. However, this is not the best way for people who are not in this type of setting to cope. Taken to extreme, this behavior can make you feel more stressed, fearful, and worn out. Instead, you should try to relax. Get plenty of rest, watch comedies, go shopping, and do fun things with your family to relieve the stress and recharge your body. You will quickly find that your body needs to recharge the mental energy that it has lost during the trauma. Even though we are suggesting you learn new ways to develop a natural sense of improved situational awareness in this book, there must be a balance between being alert to signs of danger and becoming obsessed with it. With a good sense of balance, you should feel more comfortable because you are less likely to experience harm. Conversely, if you find yourself worrying about potential danger, you should work to regain control of your life through improved balance in the way you view risk.

This book is designed to teach you ways to detect and react to danger; however, we suggest a pragmatic rather than an alarmist viewpoint not only to survive deadly encounters but also to prevent others from taking control of your life through fear. For example, we have pointed out that school violence is not as new a phenomenon as many people think, that the school homicide rate has not been skyrocketing, and that American schools often face similar security concerns as their counterparts in South Africa, England, Canada, and China. This is meant to replace fear with more accurate perspectives.

Shutting Out Reminders of the Trauma

Similar to the avoidance of people and places mentioned above, avoiding the bad memories or trying to shut out feelings is a natural reaction but can have negative impacts as well. Doing so may prevent you from confronting the overwhelming feelings and, in turn, cause you to avoid seeking help. It is important that you are able to work through the bad memories and not run from them.

In general, you should not use coping mechanisms that would have a negative long-term impact. If you have experienced significant trauma or major stressors in your life, make time to take care of yourself and get yourself out of the vortex of pain and onto a cloud of healing. If you work hard to avoid the temptation of engaging in negative coping behaviors, in time you will be able to see the long-term benefits of concentrating on yourself rather than practicing avoidance.

Once you have been able to successfully deal with your own mental health, then you can begin observing the negative coping approaches in people around you. In the beginning, just observe and contemplate. Remember, your main focus at this point is to recognize your own negative coping skills if you have any and to pull yourself out of unhealthy behavior as soon as you recognize it starting to happen. When you recognize these types of behaviors in someone else, like your child or a spouse, take the time to observe and contemplate the behavior before taking action. Focus on recognizing the behavior for what it is, a negative stress coping approach.

If you happen to observe these types of destructive patterns in others, it is important to remember to remain calm and not allow this damaging mindset to pull you into the OODA loop of bad behavior. If you can recognize these patterns in yourself and others, you can save valuable time and anguish during the healing process.

Research tells us that this is a critical point. We now know that of all military personnel who served in combat, those who were diagnosed with post traumatic stress disorder showed more avoidance, wishful thinking, and self-blame in their coping methods and fewer problem-faced coping strategies than those who reported no psychological distress (Sutker et al., 1995).

Positive Coping Strategies—What You Really Need

Most people cope successfully with 98 percent of their stressors. We make hundreds of adjustments each day and manage quite well. That means a meager 2 percent of our stressors are responsible for causing us major distress. Knowing that you only have to deal with that 2 percent may help you put problems in a more manageable perspective.

No single strategy will be effective in managing all of life's challenges, so it is imperative that you use a variety of coping skills. Most people use three or four favorite coping aids over and over again. As long as these coping skills are positive, effective, rationally applied, and not overused, any number or combination is fine. Do what works for you and your loved ones. Here are some popular coping strategies that may bring you positive results in your day-to-day life. There are some complex ways to respond to stress during a crisis, but the following can be used to create a bedrock of strong and positive mental health. This will make it easier for you to adapt to crisis stress, since your starting stress level will be lower, and you will be able to respond more effectively to the crisis in general.

"Laughter, the Best Medicine"

As Brian L. Seaward aptly states in his book, *Stressed Is Desserts Spelled Backwards,* using humor as a coping strategy can have positive effects on your mental health (Seaward, 1999). You have probably heard the old adage that laughing is the best medicine. Today we know that this is more than just a popular column in *Reader's*

Digest—there is actually research to support that claim. Melinda Smith, M.A., and Jeanne Segal, Ph.D., state: "Laughter is a powerful antidote to stress, pain, and conflict. Nothing works faster or more dependably to bring your mind and body back into balance than a good laugh" (Helpguide.org, 2013). They also note that there are tangible physical health benefits to laughter. Even the military uses humor to help soldiers deal with the stressful conditions of war. Researchers at the California-based Naval Center for Combat & Operational Stress Control (NCCOSC) noted that the military hosts USO comedy shows, events and acts geared toward making service members laugh as a way to reduce combat stress. Perhaps Bob Hope and the many other USO entertainers who have performed over the years helped do something far more important than to simply entertain so many of our troops than many of us realized. Their generosity is another example of how some people rise to the occasion to help make the best of difficult situations like war.

Here are a few other benefits of laughter:

- reduces emotional turmoil and anxiety,
- redirects negative thoughts,
- increases energy levels,
- provides ability to see serious situations from a lighter perspective,
- counters overwhelming feelings, and
- helps you focus on the important tasks at hand by making serious situations less threatening.

Exercise

Exercise is another great stress reliever. Besides the obvious medical benefits, maintaining a good workout regimen is an excellent coping mechanism. As a matter of fact, the American Council on Exercise suggests that one of the most effective methods of stress relief is exercise. The National Heart, Lung and Blood Association endorses exercise as a major activity to reduce stress and recommends that you perform any cardiovascular exercise that elevates the heart rate for 15–30 minutes, repeating the exercise at least three to four times per week.

Exercise also provides an outlet for negative emotions like irritability, frustration, and even anger. It promotes a more positive attitude and a healthier point of view, which improves your disposition by creating positive biochemical changes in the brain and body. A regular exercise routine can help reduce the amount of adrenal hormones your body releases as a counter response to stress. Furthermore, with exercise, your body releases greater amounts of endorphins, which are powerful, pain-relieving, mood-elevating chemicals in the brain (McGovern, 2005). Endorphins are natural painkillers and can also help revitalize your mood. It has been found that depressed people often lack adequate amounts of endorphins (Babyak et al., 2000).

At this point, you are probably thinking, "What types of exercise are best for relieving stress?" The answer to that question is the type of exercise you enjoy the most. A pragmatic approach to choosing a physical activity is to pick something that will keep you engaged for the long term. If you feel like the exercise is tedious, then you may not stick with it. Do what you find enjoyable. Variety is the spice of life, so mix it up from time to time. Walk, swim, run, or dance— just move. Of course, you should consult with your doctor before beginning any sort of serious exercise regimen, as there can be risks associated with exercise.

Healthy Eating

Eating is another common stress reaction. But in order for this strategy to bring you any long-term benefit, you must use care when choosing what to eat. Be watchful about binging on fatty and sugary foods. It may feel good at first, but this can have adverse effects on your psyche as well as your physique. Diets that are high in fiber and low in saturated fat have a more positive effect on your overall mood. Scientists at the Center for Health Promotion at the Johns Hopkins School of Medicine warn against meals with high-fat, high-glycemic content, which can make you feel physically dysfunctional afterward.

In particular, they note that B vitamins, especially folic acid and vitamin B12, are known to help prevent a wide range of mood disorders, including depression. These vitamins are found in spinach, romaine lettuce, lean chicken breasts, meats, fish, poultry, and dairy products (Roberts, 2010).

Remember that stress may weaken your immune system and increase your body's need for certain nutrients. A balanced diet will help keep you focused, alert, energetic, and healthy during times of stress. Conversely, a diet consisting of mostly fast food or frequently skipped meals will most likely result in poor performance or increased illnesses during stressful times. As we saw in the movie *Super Size Me,* a daily regimen of this type of food can only go on for so long before you feel worse and find yourself getting sick more often (Spurlock and Spurlock, 2004). So stay away from the junk foods and alcoholic beverages. Instead, do all you can to maintain a healthful lifestyle; your brain needs as much good fuel as possible to get you through an emotional storm. Use these natural tools that often cost nothing because they can be integrated as part of your regular diet. Remember, you are what you eat!

Talking It Out

Talking about your feelings or the situation or just having a conversation with someone you trust can do wonders to help alleviate stress. Sharing your burden can often help to lighten the load, and finding someone to talk things through as well as discuss your issues can often promote a far more upbeat and positive feeling (Giltay and Kromhout, 2006).

Bottling things up and letting the stress fester is the worst thing that you can do, as this fails to solve anything and simply enhances the stress. It is important to try to keep the conversation in a positive tone. Negative talk can have adverse effects on your psyche and can sometimes make matters worse. So when you are talking it out, use positive words and keep a positive outlook.

According to researchers at the Mayo Clinic, positive talk can promote the following benefits (Creagan, 2011):

- increased life span,
- lower rates of depression,
- lower levels of distress,
- greater resistance to the common cold,
- better psychological and physical well-being,
- reduced risk of death from cardiovascular disease, and
- better coping skills during hardships and times of stress.

Sex

We are fairly certain that you did not expect this book to tell you that sex could help you survive. However, there is research to show how even sex can be a survival mechanism. For consenting adults, sex can help relieve stress. Simon Rego, Psy.D., supervising psychologist at the Adult Outpatient Clinic of Montefiore Medical Center wrote:

> First, you have to separate the stressor from the stress reaction. So can sexual intercourse help you deal with stressors in life: conflicts at work, traffic jams? Absolutely not. But can sexual intercourse help you to feel less stressed? There's good evidence to suggest that is the case. Now that being said, there's nothing magic about sexual intercourse *per se* to relieve stress. It actually seems to be a combination of other factors that we use to create stress relief in general. Things like deeper breathing, physical exertion, touch, the release of endorphins, social connectedness. All of which can be found in other arenas, but all of which seem to come together in a sexual encounter (Rego, 2008).

Keeping in mind the limitations noted above, this example of a coping mechanism does show that there are a surprising number of strategies people can use to survive deadly encounters and to thrive in life afterward. More so, this is a perfect example of a coping mechanism that could be either positive or negative depending on how it is used.

Strategies for the Recovery Phase

Getting through the stressful times, particularly after a crisis, is called the recovery period. This phase of a crisis focuses on reducing the long-term emotional effects of a crisis. In *The Three Elements of Recovery*, the International Critical Incident Stress Foundation explains that recovery from disaster involves a physical, emotional, and spiritual rebuilding. This rebuilding process has been translated into a formula that mental health professionals can use to help survivors: talk, tears, and time (Myers and Zunin, 1990).

Talk

Two of the biggest myths in our society are "If you don't talk about it, it will go away" and "Talking about it only keeps the problem present in your mind." Too often, people feel that "no one else can understand" or that they have worn out their support systems by talking too much about their pain. But it is through talking that you will find out you are not alone and possibly help yourself and others.

Many people are frightened to talk things through because they think that discussing their problems is a sign of weakness. However, it is actually the complete opposite—talking demonstrates that you are willing to find solutions that work, that you are prepared to look at all options, and that you are not too proud to ask for help in a time of crisis.

Talking about the issues and problems that are causing you stress is a healthy and effective way of channeling your emotions and promoting a far more positive outlook through a network of support and understanding. This support will help to remedy any feelings of isolation and can help to reduce stress levels considerably (Seaward, 2012).

246

Tears

Recovery entails grief (Janoff–Bulman, 1985). Grief is the healing process by which individuals and the community gain closure from a major loss, including the apparent destruction of our assumptions about the world that we know (Myers, 1993). Tears are an essential and natural part of the psychological healing and cleansing process. As Myers puts it, "We put out fires on the hillsides relatively quickly compared to the fires that burn within our hearts. Tears are the water that quench fires of grief."

Seneca, the Roman philosopher, political leader, and author of tragedies, said: "It is sweet to mingle tears with fears; grief, where they wound in solitude, wound more deeply." His words emphasize the importance of both tears and talk in recovery as well as the importance of community during the recovery process (Smith, 2007).

Time

Time provides an opportunity for reflection and allows people to look back and recognize the challenges they have overcome. By the one-year anniversary of a disaster, most people can look inward and appreciate the courage, stamina, endurance, resourcefulness, and growth they have found within themselves and each other. They can look around and appreciate the loved ones and friends who have helped them through the healing. At an anniversary, most people no longer see themselves as "victims," but as "survivors" with a great deal to look forward to (Myers, 1994b).

Dealing with Acute Crisis Stress

Every day we make choices that affect our lives sometimes for many years to come. In the summer of 2007, a young woman made a decision to meet someone in person whom she had been communicating with on the Internet. She felt isolated and wanted to connect with somebody. This man in particular seemed to understand her personality. They were only going to hang out and talk as friends.

She felt proud that she was able to reach out and socialize. Nervous and excited, she arrived at his address. When he greeted her at the door, she immediately noticed that the apartment seemed to have been decorated by an older woman rather than the young man who lived there alone. He had also clearly been drinking, but she ignored her intuition since she was trying to be more outgoing and meet new friends.

This visit was not entirely reckless. After all, they had been friends for several months, with conversations growing more and more personal as many close friendships are bound to. After months of talking online, she had confided in him that her personality was asexual in nature because she had been molested as a child. He had seemed very understanding. He had not treated her differently as others had. Now, sitting in his living room and talking in person, she continued to talk openly about her personal history. She was vulnerable, and he knew it. As he hugged her to offer comfort, she felt uncomfortable, and she told him to stop, but he dismissed her as being hypersensitive.

Just as de Becker describes in the *Gift of Fear*, this attacker showed the early warning sign of ignoring the word "No." The encounter quickly became more violent as he brutally raped and sodomized her for more than an hour using the full weight of his body to hold her captive. She felt stunned as though what was happening was in a movie. She was finally able to scream, which stunned him for a second and allowed her a chance to escape. As she ran to her car and sped off in terror, she could only hear the sounds of laughter from the monster that took so much from her that night. He laughed away her dignity, her respect, her trust, her body, and her peace of mind.

This story happened to one of the staff members who helped work on this book, but it is hardly unique. Unfortunately, many women experience this type of encounter at some point in their lives. Every two minutes a sexual assault takes place in the United States, and 38 percent of rapists are acquaintances of the victim (RAINN.org, 2009).

When she reported her case to the police, she endured a legal process that seemed to last an eternity, including threats that her friends would be interviewed by private investigators seeking information to discredit her. She also endured the shame and blame of her friends who told her that she should have known better. As a final insult, the prosecutor eventually advised that she should probably drop the charges unless she was comfortable with her personal life being paraded in front of her family in the courtroom as the defense counsel tried to discredit her. She had already gone through the embarrassing process of evidence collection as strangers had examined and taken photos of her naked body to show the bruising and internal injuries as proof of a brutal crime. She had recounted the story of that night over and over again to investigators, prosecutors, social workers, family, friends, and others in pursuit of justice. She now lives with the memory of that night forever etched in her mind. In this case, the victim was met with a less than desirable response from public safety. Thankfully, most public safety, mental health, and prosecution professionals work diligently so the challenges this woman faced can be lessened. If you find yourself in this type of situation, be sure to make sure you have all the facts available to you and you have adequate legal representation.

Although the aforementioned coping strategies can help create the bedrock of mental wellness that will help you respond and recover from a crisis, handling the immediate stress of a crisis like this one can be much more demanding of a nuanced approach. We have discussed a number of simple practices throughout this book that can help you deal with acute crisis stress during your immediate response. Practicing controlled breathing, using mental simulation, and starting out with a positive mindset of survival can all help before or during the crisis. It is also important to consider these same topics in the context of recovery from a traumatic or life-changing event. Survivors of extreme trauma often feel dissociated from the world. As one concentration camp survivor put it, "We did not yet belong to this world" when survivors were rescued by American troops. However, even though it is nearly impossible to live life without experiencing trauma, we are also inherently equipped to focus on survival strategies so that we can move on and live our lives (Gonzalez, 2012).

In addition to traditional counseling services, there are several accepted models for mental health crisis response for incidents of acute crisis stress. If you are a decision maker or crisis responder in an organization, it is important to understand these models and choose one for use in your recovery efforts. It can also be helpful for the average person to understand these models since you may encounter this type of process if you experience a major crisis event. It is important to understand that these models are simply examples of popular types of crisis intervention activities, and this list is not all-inclusive.

Among the various crisis response models, the International Critical Incident Stress Foundation (ICISF) model is one of the most widely used around the world. The ICISF model is called Critical Incident Stress Management, or CISM/CISD (Critical Incident Stress Management/Critical Incident Stress Debriefing). There are other popular recovery models in each country. In the United States, the two most widely used recovery models are the National Organization for Victim's Assistance (NOVA) and National Association of School Psychologists (NASP) model. There are a few other models including those used by the American Red Cross and other organizations dedicated to helping those in crisis. The primary goal of each model and technique is to allow for the ventilation and validation of feelings in order to prevent long-term harmful impact of a disaster on your psyche. In essence, the models are to help reduce the overwhelming feelings of helplessness and hopelessness that you may encounter when dealing with a crisis.

In addition to these recognized models that crisis responders and mental health professionals use to heal others, these same healers must also protect themselves. It can be incredibly easy for someone in these roles to focus so much on helping others that he or she can be personally overwhelmed by crisis stress. Coauthor Sonayia Shepherd has experienced compassion fatigue when responding to a crisis and can attest firsthand to the importance of taking a step back and evaluating yourself from time to time. The models above can also be applied to first responders, and one that is particularly well suited for this purpose is the CISM model described above (Brookes, 2009).

There is an entire branch of therapy dedicated to helping people recover from a traumatic event. Tina Brookes, Ed.D., is a licensed clinical social worker with over 20 years of experience as a professional educator and mental health professional. In this dual role, she has provided crisis response intervention to incidents both in her home state and around the world, including the Aurora Colorado shootings and the Sandy Hook tragedy. She also trains all kinds of people on these topics, from students in her hometown to decision makers around the country.

Tina recounts a story in which she was visiting a small village in Brazil when she was asked to counsel a young girl who had been raped. She uses this story as an example of how quickly a person can be drawn into a crisis. In this case she was in the middle of breakfast and had to respond immediately. She had to adapt to the local conditions and the use of a translator who happened to be a 20-year-old male. Tina had to work hard to overcome a language barrier and adverse conditions to provide the same advice she would give the woman in the previous story: she is not to blame for what happened to her, she is not "damaged goods" or deserving of shame or guilt, and she should avoid keeping her emotions and reactions buried (Brookes, 2013).

This is not to ignore the potential to prevent violence and the need for victims to learn from their experiences. In fact, past experience can be one of the best teachers. Rather, the point is that emotional survival can be just as important as physical survival. For more about dealing with traumatic crisis stress, visit *www.SafeHavensInternational.org.*

Children and Traumatic Stress

Children are not exempt from feeling the pangs of stress. Being exposed to traumatic situations can obviously cause severe stress reactions in youngsters. Exposure can come in a variety of forms, like actually being in a crisis, seeing traumatic scenes on television, and even overhearing adults having discussions about a crisis event. It is important that you try to limit a child's exposure when going through a stressful situation. That may mean turning off the television and taking a break from the news. This does not mean censoring information or trying to shelter a child from reality—rather it is critical that we understand the need to limit the impact of the modern phenomenon of information saturation as part of the 24-hour news cycle.

During the September 11 terrorist attacks, Dr. Shepherd responded to numerous phone calls from schools asking if it is prudent to allow students to watch the events and the aftermath unfold as part of social studies or current event classes. As she advised educators then, parents should be careful about exposing children to too much sadness and horror even if it is in the interest of learning. People do not have to be directly involved in an event to start exhibiting traumatic stress reactions. Hearing an event or seeing it on television can easily cause stress for a person, especially those who are still in the various stages of adolescent development.

There are a number of things you can do to help a child or teen who might be stressed by crisis events, or even just the child's school, family, or friends. The first thing that is most important is to talk to the child or teen to find out what might be triggering the child's stress. It is important to find out whether the stress might be caused by external factors like a heavy schedule, a heavy workload and/or course load, or relationship drama. The situation may also be caused by something deeper, for example if the child is having trouble coping or does not have enough coping skills in his or her arsenal so that the child can tackle the stress the child is dealing with.

Once you have talked to the child and have a basic understanding of the issues at hand, then you can make suggestions or adjustments, either addressing the external factors that are causing stress or helping improve the child's coping skills. This might be accomplished by learning new coping techniques and new ways to relax or learning better strategies to handle the situations that are creating stress in the child's life. In severe cases, you may even look at changing a school or work schedule and even considering having the child see a therapist or a counselor for some help.

Despite your best efforts, children are sometimes exposed to crisis events. If that happens, you must help the child cope according to his or her developmental abilities and make sure that your approach is age appropriate. The Centers for Disease Control and Prevention (CDC) created a fact sheet for caregivers who help children cope. The document, titled *Parents Helping Youth Cope with Disaster* highlights the following points:

- **Maintain a normal routine.** Helping children wake up, go to sleep, and eat meals at regular times provides them a sense of stability. Going to school and participating in typical after-school activities also provides stability and extra support.

- **Talk, listen, and encourage expression.** Create opportunities to encourage your children to talk, but do not force them. Listen to your child's thoughts and feelings and share some of your own. After a traumatic event, it is important for children to feel like they can share their feelings and to know that their fears and worries are understandable. Keep these conversations going by asking them how they feel in a week, then in a month, and so on.

- **Watch and listen.** Be alert for any change in behavior. Are children sleeping more or less than usual? Are they withdrawing from friends or family? Are they behaving in any way out of the ordinary? Any changes in behavior, even small changes, may be signs that the child is having trouble coming to terms with the event and may need support.

- **Reassure.** Stressful events can challenge a child's sense of physical and emotional safety and security. Take opportunities to reassure your child about his or her safety and well-being and discuss ways that you, the school, and the community are taking steps to keep your child safe.
- **Connect with others.** Make it an ongoing effort to talk to other parents and your child's teachers about concerns and ways to help your child cope. You do not have to deal with problems alone. It is often helpful for parents, schools, and health professionals to work together to support and ensure the well-being of all children in stressful times (CDC, 2013).

It is also important to remind children that it is okay to cry, even for boys. In some cultures, men are respected more if they cry, and they are sometimes even expected to cry. Sometimes, a good cry is therapeutic and does wonders for the mind, body, and soul.

Whether or not you are helping yourself, your child, or your community, it is important to remember that positive coping mechanisms can make all the difference.

Conclusion

In the story at the beginning of this chapter, Mrs. Abi and her daughter found themselves grieving together as they coped with the loss of a precious life they once knew. But with the help of professional counseling, family support systems, and their faith, they were able to make it through, and their family grew even tighter.

After the brutal rape that we described earlier in this chapter, the young woman carried the baggage of her experience in every encounter from that night onward. Between the harassing messages from her attacker and the seemingly pervasive threat of repeated sexual assault from others, her life was filled with fear. She was jumpy, and the nightmares seemed relentless. To this day, she is still unable to remember a good part of a year of her life because she had to numb herself to the outside world to keep going on. But with time, patience, and a plethora of support, she was able to smile again. She was able to work her way though the web of hurt and pain through the help she received from family and friends. Finally, she was also able to do something she never thought she could do—form a meaningful bond with someone of the opposite sex. Today she is in a loving relationship and is able to share her horrific story to inspire other women who have gone through similar situations and let them know that they are not alone. More importantly, her story reminds us that we always have to listen to our gut instincts, watch for the warning signs of danger, and avoid the trap of denial. She was not alone in this story in ignoring the warning signs of danger, as her friends later said things like "I had a bad feeling but I didn't want to offend you." It is important for friends and loved ones to speak out when they see something that bothers them.

Whether the result of stress-related medical issues or mental health concerns, the stress of a major event can kill you even though you managed to survive an event. Whether you die from a gunman's bullet or a heart attack or because you take your own life as a response to traumatic events you survive, death is death. On the other hand, we can take stressful situations and turn them into a positive experience that results in growth and personal development beyond what we previously thought even possible. You do have an astounding amount of control over how stress affects you. You will have stress if you survive a life and death situation, but this does not automatically mean that stress must have control over you.

Key Points in Chapter Fifteen

- It is crucial that you try to get out and rejoin society after a crisis.
- Avoiding the bad memories or trying to shut out feelings is a natural reaction, which may cause you to avoid seeking help. It is important that you are able to work through bad memories and not run from them.
- You should not use coping mechanisms that would have a negative long-term impact.

- Make time to take care of yourself, and then you can begin observing and addressing negative coping approaches in people around you.
- Recognize your own negative coping skills to pull yourself out of unhealthy behavior as soon as you recognize it starting to happen.
- As little as 2 percent of our stressors are responsible for causing us major distress.
- There are tangible physical health benefits to laughter.
- Maintaining a good workout regimen is an excellent coping mechanism, and it also provides an outlet for negative emotions like irritability, frustration, and even anger.
- Endorphins are natural painkillers, which can also help revitalize your mood. It has been found that depressed people often lack adequate amounts of endorphins.
- Diets that are high in fiber and low in saturated fat have a more positive effect on your overall mood.
- Stress may weaken your immune system and increase your body's need for certain nutrients.
- A conversation with appropriate trusted individuals can do wonders to help alleviate stress. Talking demonstrates that you are willing to find solutions that work.
- Negative talk can have adverse effects on your psyche and can sometimes make matters worse.
- Crying is an essential and natural part of the psychological healing and cleansing process. A good cry is therapeutic and does wonders for the mind, body, and soul.
- Time provides an opportunity for reflection.
- People do not have to be directly involved in an event to start exhibiting traumatic stress reactions.

BIBLIOGRAPHY

Anspaugh, D. J., M. H. Hamrick, and F. D. Rosato (2006). *Wellness: Concepts and applications.* New York: McGraw-Hill.

Babyak, M., J. A. B., S. Herman, P. Khatri, M. Doraiswamy, K. Moore, E. Craighead, T. T. Baldewicz, and K. R. Krishnan. (2000). Exercise treatment for major depression: Maintenance of therapeutic benefit at 10 months. *Psychosomatic Medicine, 62*(5), 633–638.

Brookes, T. (2009). *Critical incident stress management services.* Triad Regional Advisory Council, North Carolina.

Brookes, T. (2013). The power of preparedness in crisis response. *Grief, Crisis & Disaster Network, 1* (1).

CDC: *Parents helping youth cope with disaster.* (2013). Atlanta, GA: Centers for Disease Control. Retrieved from *http://www.cdc.gov/violenceprevention/pdf/coping-parents-cope-with-disaster-2013-508.pdf*

Creagan, E. (2011). *Positive talk.* Rochester, MN: Mayo Clinic.

Giltay, E., and D. Kromhout. (2006). Dispositional optimism and the risk of depressive symptoms during 15 years of follow-up: The Zutphen Elderly Study. *Journal of Affective Disorders, 91*(1), 45–52.

Gonzalez, L. (2012). *Surviving survival: The art and science of resilience.* New York: W. W. Norton & Company.

Helpguide.org. (2013). Retrieved July 15, 2013, from *http://www.helpguide.org/*

Janoff-Bulman, R. (1985). The aftermath of victimization: Rebuilding shattered assumptions. In C. R. Figley (Ed.), *Trauma and its wake, Vol. I.* New York: Brunner/Mazel.

Janoff-Bulman, R.; I H. F. (1983). A theoretical perspective for understanding reactions to victimization. *Journal of Social Issues, 39*(2), 1–17.

McGovern, M. (2005). The effects of exercise on the brain. Retrieved July 15, 2013, from *http://serendip.brynmawr.edu/bb/neuro/neuro05/web2/mmcgovern.html*

Meyers, D., and L. M. Zunin. (1990). Talk, tears and time. *Today's Supervisors, 6*(11), 14–15.

Myers, D. (1994a). Psychological recovery from disaster: Key concepts for delivery of mental health services. *NCP Clinical Quarterly, 4*(2).

Myers, D. (1994b). The anniversary of the disaster: Mental health issues and interventions *Disaster response and recovery: A handbook for mental health professionals.* Rockville, MD: Center for Mental Health Services.

Myers, D. (1993, May 14). The healing continues. Paper presented at the Disaster: Partners in Response and Recovery Conference, San Bernadino, CA.

Negative coping and PTSD. (December 20, 2011). Retrieved July 22, 2013, from *http://www.ptsd.va.gov/public/pages/ptsd-negative-coping.asp*

Statistics: RAINN: Rape, Abuse & Incest National Network. Rape, Abuse & Incest National Network, 2009. Retrieved September 15th, 2013 at *www.rainn.org.*

Rego, S. (2008). Can having sexual intercourse help me deal with stress? *ABC News.* Retrieved from *http://abcnews.go.com/Health/StressCoping/story?id=4673725#.UeS3alOvt7Z*

Roberts, S., and R. Tranter. (2010). Half-baked? B vitamins and depression. *The American Journal of Clinical Nutrition, 92*(2), 269–270. doi: 10.3945/ajcn.2010.29977

Seaward, B. L. (1999). *Stressed is desserts spelled backwards: Rising above life's challenges with humor, hope and courage.* Berkeley, CA: Conari Press.

Seaward, B. L. (2012). *Managing stress: Principles and strategies for health and well-being* (7th ed.). Burlington, MA: Jones & Bartlett Learning.

Smith, W. (Ed.) (2007). London, England: I. B. Tauris.

Spurlock, M. (Writer) & M. Spurlock (Director). (2004). *Super Size Me* [Film]. In M. Spurlock (Producer): Samuel Goldwin Films.

Statistics: RAINN: Rape, Abuse & Incest National Network. (2009). Rape, Abuse & Incest National Network. Retrieved September 15, 2013, from *www.rainn.org*

Sutker, P., J. J. V., K. Brailey, and A. N. Allain. (1995). Memory, attention, and executive deficits in POW survivors: Contributing biological and psychological factors. *Neuropsychology, 9*(1), 118–125.

CHAPTER SIXTEEN

WORDS CAN HURT

Sticks and stones can break our bones, but words can hurt survivors.

Erin and Abe were beginning to get their life back to a "new normal" after the attack on their home on April 29, 2013. Abe's physical wounds were healing, and after a couple of weeks, he was able to bring himself to enter his own home. Coauthor Steve Satterly and his wife went to Abe's home to help his wife Erin clean the blood off of what seemed like everything in the house. It seemed that Erin and Abe were making a natural progression through the emotional healing process.

But on June 14, 2013, their attacker was released from jail and placed on home detention. Knowing that their attacker was out of jail created near panic in both Erin and Abe. After their violent experience the last time they encountered him, they were not willing to bet their lives that the attacker would abide by the home arrest restrictions. Their situation was exacerbated by the fact that their attacker, a pharmacist, was allowed to go back to work, to work at a pharmacy that Erin would possibly have to visit as part of her student rotations.

What was worse was that the attacker's father attempted to contact them. A university assistant dean provided the father with the e-mail addresses of friends and acquaintances of his son, who was a third-year medical student. Soon, the father was e-mailing the attacker's friends, acquaintances of Erin and Abe's, with his son's version of the story, a version that painted Erin and Abe as interlopers who overreacted to the situation with unjustified violence. The father told the friends that when his son was in the hospital prior to the incident, his wife had not been there for him. He also asked these friends for money to help make his son's bail. These people, whom the couple had considered friends, started sending messages that conveyed that the couple were overreacting to what had happened and that pressing charges was an unfair response. Erin and Abe felt victimized all over again.

More than any time, this is when Erin and Abe needed support from family and friends to recover. This is one reason why receiving the opposite reaction—accusation and second-guessing—can be so damaging, especially when it comes from friends. The friends might not have intentionally meant to hurt Erin and Abe again, but they did. Instead of helping Erin and Abe, their friends, intentionally or accidentally, made it even more difficult for them to recover. In the previous chapter, we discussed how a person facing a crisis could cope to overcome the situation. In this chapter, we will examine what family, friends, and society should do to help their loved ones, friends, or anyone who is in the process of recovery from a crisis. After all, Abe and Eric did recover. So how can you?

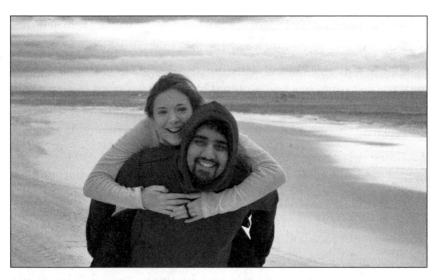

Abe and Erin: Abe and Erin are college students who survived a deadly encounter by acting fast when a man with a hatchet and two hammers suddenly burst into their home and started attacking them. Their story is an important example of how friends and community can be a helpful—or harmful—piece of the recovery process.
Photo: personal collection of Abhigya Singh

How to Talk to Someone Who Is Facing a Crisis

Sticks and stones can break my bones, but words will never hurt me. This is a common phrase that most of us have uttered at one time or another. But this old adage is not always true. Words do matter, and they can hurt, especially people who have survived a tragedy. They can also hurt those who have lost loved ones in a crisis. This is true even when no harm is intended. Surviving a crisis incident requires plenty of physical and emotional support, which includes saying the right things.

Knowing what to say to someone who is going through a crisis is not an innate ability. People must be taught how to use words wisely. What you say can determine the outcome of a crisis as much as your actions. Whether it is giving directions or comforting a friend, your communication can have lasting effects.

There is a saying, "Burdens shared with a friend are often lighter to carry." Discussing your troubles with someone is a way of expressing emotions and can help get rid of some of their effects, too. Putting feelings into words can help a person see the situation more objectively. Sometimes, just knowing someone is aware of our feelings, worries, or difficult responsibilities can positively impact our emotional state after a stressful event.

Conversely, knowing what to say to someone in a crisis is equally important. One of the most important things to remember is not to give false hope. People in trouble desperately want to be reassured, and all of your emotions may urge you to give that reassurance. However, a "there, there, everything will be all right" approach may actually be a disservice—everything may not be all right. By giving false hope, you may be relegating the troubled person to the status of a child, with no control and not even a stake in the process, making the person feel weaker. Instead of unrealistic comfort, a statement of faith that he or she will be strong enough to survive is a more appropriate strategy. Help the person help himself. Let the person know you are available to help find a solution. Lend a shoulder as an equal, instead of reassuring him or her like a parent.

This provides a more important kind of reassurance—that you have faith in the troubled person's ability to handle the crisis. Reassuring children is critical when facing a crisis and may require customized approaches based on the situation. Children typically crave positive attention when they have been propelled into a crisis event. So provide it for them. They may need to be reminded that it is okay to cry, or they may want to hold your hand.

The following strategies can help you say the right thing when a person is going through a crisis. These types of techniques can be applied to children or adults. There are many different ways to let a person know you care, but some of us get tongue-tied when dealing with individuals going through a traumatic event, and the following strategies are accepted by experts throughout the field of crisis intervention.

Establish a Rapport

A crisis state can make a person feel like no one can understand the situation. An event can be even more upsetting when a survivor encounters this frustration. To defeat this cycle, it is important to win the person's trust. This can be done through a technique called validation. For example, instead of saying, "I understand," use indirect acknowledgment by validating what the person is feeling and redirecting that into words. Saying, "I'd certainly be upset too," or, "That must be frustrating. You have every right to be angry," shows empathy and validates that person's feeling without being condescending. Unless you have gone through the exact same crisis, you cannot understand what that particular person is going through so do not pretend you do.

Develop an Action Plan

Once you have enough information, you can help the person in crisis explore options, both in the current instance and for the future. It is important to avoid a response that blames the person for what happened. Do not say, "Next time, you should evacuate sooner," for example. Build a plan for moving forward. The more concrete the plan, the better. Include tasks the person in crisis can focus on to improve the situation. Exploring alternatives and finding a path to a solution helps a person get through the short-term state of a crisis.

What Not to Say

Just like knowing what to say, knowing what *not* to say to a person in a crisis is equally important. While properly talking to a person facing a crisis can aid in the recovery process, inappropriate wording can make the situation worse, thus doing more harm than good. A simple slip of the tongue or inappropriate laugh can have dramatic effects. The example of saying "I know how you feel" is another time when good intentions can backfire. Unfortunately, we are often prone to say things like this because we have heard this ourselves so many times after a tragedy.

Do not mislead the distressed person. When helping a person in crisis, avoid telling him or her that everything is okay when you know it is not. Doing so will break that trust and could prompt another crisis. As important as it is to reach out, it is equally important to understand what your role is. It is very tempting when confronted with someone else's pain to try and fix it. It is likely that the person is already getting lots of advice from other sources, including suggestions from qualified professionals. So the best thing you can often do is to listen and let the person know that you hear his or her pain. This is especially important in the wake of a break-up or divorce where there are often dual, and commonly, dueling, narratives as to what actually happened. As a side note, this is also particularly good advice for raising children. Most of the time you should listen to their problems and acknowledge their hurt—no matter how absurd it may sound—rather than telling them what to do.

In addition, no matter how frustrated you are at a person's mental state, never tell a stressed person, "Come on, snap out of it," or, "Some people have it much worse than you." You would not tell a person with asthma or diabetes to snap out of it would you? In this context, depression and stress should be viewed in the same light. Asking someone to "just snap out of it" or "just be happy" makes that person feel inadequate or that the person is doing something wrong. Furthermore, comparing an individual's circumstances to people who are suffering greater hardship is of no use either.

Statements like these also confront sufferers with their situation and put pressure on them. This can cause the sufferers to retreat further and further into their own world. The best thing to do is to offer love and support, for example, by saying, "I'm always here if you need me or want to talk." And three little words can mean so much: "I love you," if they are appropriate and the person hearing them knows they are sincere (Shields and Somerville, 1994).

In addition, people in crisis should be allowed to feel whatever they are expressing to you, and you should never tell someone in crisis how to feel, nor should you say, "You need to calm down." It is important to note that when emotions are high, you are the one who should remain calm. Try to speak in a calm, even voice. This is not always easy if someone is yelling at you. Just take deep breaths and focus on speaking calmly. Doing so will often project a balanced example, and this calm demeanor can help to relax the person you are talking to.

The Power of Positive Words

As a loved one, friend, or community partner, it is totally natural to want to understand what is happening to a friend who is suffering from stress. There is nothing wrong with that if it is done appropriately. However, a problem can arise if you start to impose your knowledge on the person instead of offering comfort. This can happen when you observe certain behaviors and habits exhibited by the person and comment on why they are behaving in such a way. For example, if you hear a victim put him- or herself down, you could say, "That's a part of your illness. I've been reading about it, and self-deprecation is one of the reasons why people become depressed. You need to stop putting yourself down." This approach is confrontational and may in turn put the sufferer under pressure, which may cause the sufferer to dismiss your comments and withdraw socially because of the fear that he or she is being scrutinized.

A more effective response is to very gently remind the sufferer of a time when he or she did something good or achieved a success. For example, if you hear a person say, "I'm useless, I never get anything right." You can say "Sure you do, hey, remember the time when you…." Do you see the difference in approach? The first is more like a doctor assessing a patient; the second is just a normal, natural conversation and does not mention stress, depression, or anxiety. This is a more helpful response since it shifts the focus from a negative emotion ("I'm useless…") to a good one ("remember when…") without exerting pressure.

Positive words can often lead to a positive outlook, which ends with positive results. Keep an optimistic attitude around those who are dealing with difficult emotions by using positive words and a positive tone. If you are unsure about what to say, there is an array of resources that can help. For example, Hallmark has a website devoted to the subject of positive words (Dubin, 2013). Visit *http://www.hallmark.com/encouragement/ideas/comforting-words/* for more information.

The Art of Listening

Similar to positive words, being a good listener can also lend significant positive support to a person in the recovery phase of a crisis. Give the person space and time, and let the person tell his or her story. Be an active listener, which means making sure the person knows you are part of the conversation by asking questions and injecting verbal cues, like "Uh huh" and "I see." Another technique is repeating to someone what they just said to you. For example, if they say, "I'm upset I lost my home," respond with "So you're upset that you lost your house. I'd be upset too." People commonly feel better if they can tell their story to a listening ear.

You should also listen for warning signs of risky behavior. Be alert for certain words and phrases that might indicate a person is in profound distress. Statements like "This is hopeless" or "My life is over" are indicators that a person is in crisis and may need a referral for professional assistance or long-term care. If you feel that the person is contemplating hurting him- or herself or others, report the situation to authorities and/or a suicide hotline. You may need to ask the person directly, "Are you considering suicide?" Whether you face a major life event or the loss of a loved one, it is crucial to ask. Remember, if a person is not thinking about it, most likely he or she will say no. And if the person is, the fact that someone asked to talk about it will be a relief and a release for a person in crisis. Helping someone after a crisis is not about removing the symptoms but identifying the underlying causes to prevent problems in the future.

When helping people through a time of crisis, remind them of the first rule in a crisis: do not make a bad situation worse by adopting permanent solutions to a temporary problem. For example, suicide is one common permanent solution to a temporary problem. Depending on the context, quitting a job or moving away are other, less life-threatening examples of drastic responses to crisis stress. Make sure they understand that they have better options if the situation seems dire (Bornstein, 2006).

If the person is going to talk it out, you must be a good listener. Good listening encourages people to talk about their problems. Here are key strategies for active listening:

- Stop talking. You cannot listen if you are talking.
- Initiate and maintain eye contact with the person. If you are going to listen to someone, look at him or her. Vary eye contact rather than staring fixedly or with undue intensity.
- Put yourself in the other person's place. Recalling how you might have felt in a similar situation or how others were affected might help. Do not assume, however, that the person's responses will be or should be the same as yours.

- To help the person get started, use open-ended questions that cannot be answered with "yes" or "no." This will allow the person to go into the subject at length. Some examples of open-ended questions or statements are:
  - "Tell me about _____."
  - "Would you like to talk about _____?"
  - "Let's discuss _____."
- Show you are paying attention. Relax your body, and let your movements be natural. For example, if you usually gesture a lot or make a lot of jokes, feel free to do so now in a manner fitting the situation.
- Take your cue for your next response or action from what the person is saying. Do not focus on covering your agenda, jump from subject to subject, or interrupt. If you cannot think of anything to say, go back to something the person said earlier and ask a question about that. There is no need to talk about yourself or offer your opinion.
- Once you've encouraged the person to talk, your response can make a big difference in keeping the conversation going. Remember to nod your head, interject with short, encouraging statements like, "Oh?" or "Then what happened?" In response to a statement, try saying things like:
  - "Tell me more."
  - "How did you feel about that?"
  - "What does that mean to you?"
- Ask questions and listen to the answers. Try and find out how the person feels.
- Do not try to guess what the person is going to say, and don't answer without really listening.
- Repeat what you think the person said, asking if you are right, for example: "Is this how you feel?"
- Don't judge the person—it can stop communication.
- Don't encourage finger pointing or blaming on others.

Reassurance

Sometimes we are afraid to reach out to friends in acute crises because we think that they will be embarrassed or ashamed. At other times, we just do not want to share, either because our problems are too personal or because we are so submerged in our own issues that we cannot be physically or emotionally available. But just as it is important not to ignore physical pain in ourselves, it is equally important not to ignore emotional pain in those close to us. If a friend is contemplating suicide, for example, it is important for him to know that you do not want to live in a world that he is not part of. Many crises occur because people feel isolated and in despair. Let them know that you are there and that they matter to you. Below are some techniques to reassure somebody who is in a crisis.

Emphasize the Positive

Often, persons going through a crisis situation cannot see the positive things in life. They cannot fathom positive opportunities or see that they will overcome their situation. Pointing out the positives in their situation—the silver lining in the storm cloud—can often lead to a mental breakthrough for the better.

Send Them Something

One way to let a close friend know that you are thinking about him or her is to send the friend something thoughtful. Right after coauthor Shepherd's grandmother died, one of her friends sent her a care package filled with oils, bubble bath gels, and lotions. The friend knew that her grandmother used to send her these types of gifts in the mail regularly, and this was her friend's way of saying "I'm thinking about you." It made her day to know that someone was trying to make the day a little better for her.

But it does not always have to be a present. Dr. Shepherd often sends e-cards, thoughtful notes, or uplifting text messages to friends who are sad just to brighten their day. Depending on the personality of the person you wish to help and the specific situation, you can also send poems, song lyrics, or articles you come across that speak to the types of challenges the individual is going through. These are noninvasive ways of letting a friend know that he or she is on your mind. Sometimes a phone call just to say hello provides much comfort and calm reassurance.

Recognize Your Limitations

Perhaps the most important thing you can do is to recognize that you are not all-powerful. Dr. Shepherd recently came across this post by a friend on Facebook, and it spoke volumes to her: "I find it enormously heartbreaking to watch someone I love suffer under the weight of severe depression. I feel so useless."

It is really hard to accept, but at the end of the day, there is only so much you can do. But you can save yourself a lot of unnecessary grief if you acknowledge that you are not in control. You cannot fix this person's life. You can only show the individual love and urge him or her to seek professional assistance.

When people are in crisis, they have a tendency to become angry and blame others for the event or loss. Research shows that people who do not cope successfully with a crisis have an overwhelming tendency to dwell on the people or things they imagined were responsible for their trouble. Researcher Margarita Tartakovsky notes that blaming is a way of avoiding the truth. Instead of facing the facts, we focus on what might have been instead of looking at the problem at hand.

Do not encourage someone in trouble to speculate on the "villain" with the idea that he or she will feel better if the blame is placed on someone else. Laying blame can make it harder or less likely for the person to come out of the crisis strengthened, whether the villain is a person, a natural disaster, or a disease. Blaming can occur whether it is discouraged or not, so listen patiently and try not to fuel the blaming. Encourage the person to see the other side. It is very difficult to survive a crisis situation from under a cloud of blame (Tartakovsky, 2012).

Critical incidents will instantly reveal more about you than you ever thought possible. What you believe about life, money, love, family, honesty, courage, hope, faith, and everything else in life will surface when everything that you thought that you believed in is suddenly shaken. Know that a crisis may take you straight to the very thing that you fear the most. In some cases, this can ultimately be good because you do not have any choice other than to face it and get through the situation the best way you can. None of this is easy, but the character and maturity you develop while struggling to just get through the day will last for years. Besides talking, it can be helpful to journal out those fears and spend some time writing down what you believe during times like this. The insights you generate about your own identity can help you get through future events faster and stronger than you ever imagined. This is the process of removing fear to replace it with a deeper assurance.

Conclusion

Sometimes bad things happen to good people, and there is not much we can say to make it better. At these times, it can be best not to even try to help with words. If you feel that words would not help the situation, use your presence, help with a meal, assist with child-care, or look for other small ways to help the person focus his time and energies on coping. Offering gift certificates for nearby restaurants could help if the person is having trouble cooking or cleaning after the crisis or if the person is facing financial hardship as a result. Pitching in to help pay for a needed car repair or praying for someone you know in crisis are some other small gestures that we can make to help others who are facing difficulty.

While you may not have any real answers, this does not mean you are powerless to help. Your encouraging words of hope and your supportive actions can mean the world to someone who is feeling scared and alone. It is better to say, "Hang in there" and "I'm here to help if I can" than to retreat in silence and do nothing because you are not sure of what to say. Taking action to do something positive to help someone get through the day can be more productive than spending massive amounts of time and energy trying to figure out the answer to some of the questions that might never be answered anyway. Closing the door to all of the "what ifs" will allow your mind to open up other doors of options and possibilities. This can be true even in the most challenging of situations. Survival is predicated on finding a way to get through a bad situation emotionally and physically. Just like the measures we have talked about to help prevent, prepare for, or respond to a crisis, responding to the aftereffects of a crisis is a critical part of any long-term survival strategy.

Key Points in Chapter Sixteen

- Words do matter, and they can hurt, especially for people who have survived a tragedy.
- People must be taught how to use words wisely, since this is not an innate ability.
- What you say can determine the outcome of a crisis as much as your actions can.
- Putting feelings into words can help a person see the situation more objectively.
- People in trouble desperately want to be reassured, but it is important to remember not to give false hope.
- Lend a shoulder as an equal.
- Avoid a response that blames the person for what happened.
- Never tell someone in crisis how to feel. You also should not say, "You need to calm down." When emotions are high, you are the one that should remain calm to relax the person you are talking to.
- It is natural to want to understand what is happening to a friend who is suffering from stress.
- Try to gently remind the person of a time when he or she did something good or achieved a success. Positive words can often lead to a positive outlook, which ends with positive results.

- Being a good listener can also lend significant positive support to a person in the recovery phase of a crisis. Good listening can encourage a person to talk about problems.
- Be alert for warning signs of risky behavior.
- Do not make a bad situation worse by adopting permanent solutions to a temporary problem.
- Use noninvasive ways of letting the person know that he or she is on your mind like sending a card or gift.
- Blaming is a way of avoiding the truth. Laying blame can make it harder or less likely for the person to come out of the crisis.

BIBLIOGRAPHY

Barranti, C., and I. Service S. U. C. E. (1985). *Encouraging a friend to seek professional help.* Cooperative Extension Service, Iowa State University.

Bornstein, K. (2006). *Hello, cruel world: 101 alternatives to suicide for teens, freaks, and other outlaws.* New York: Seven Stories Press.

Dubin, J. W. (2013). I'm here for you: The right words—and actions—for life's tough times. Retrieved July 16, 2013, from *http://www.hallmark.com/encouragement/ideas/comforting-words/*

Marotz-Baden, R. (1988). *Families in rural America: Stress adaptation and revitalization.* St. Paul, MN: National Council on Family Relations.

Shields, K., and P. Somerville. (1994). In the tiger's mouth: An empowerment guide for social action; Gabriola Island: New Society.

Tartakovsky, M. (2012). 9 best ways to support someone with depression. World of Psychology. Retrieved from *http://psychcentral.com/blog/archives/2012/05/08/9-best-ways-to-support-someone-with-depression/*

CONCLUSION: LIFE IS A BLESSING

We cannot allow tragedy to destroy the joy of living.

We have discussed plenty of tragedies in this book. You could easily become overwhelmed and view the world as a more dangerous place if you take these stories out of context. We hope instead that you will remember that the world has always been a dangerous place to some extent. In most ways, we are much safer today than we were one thousand, one hundred, or even a dozen years ago.

Due to advancements in the medical field, we now routinely outlive crisis events that were almost always fatal just a few decades ago. There have been scores of magnificent advancements in safety as well. At the same time, today's technology also means that we are now more than ever painfully aware of terrible situations like the attack at Sandy Hook Elementary School.

Catastrophic school violence in the United States dates back to the first mass casualty attack where Enoch Brown and his students were massacred in 1764. Contrary to the popular belief that American schools are inherently dangerous, schools are far more dangerous in places like the People's Republic of China. During the 2008 Sichuan Earthquake, 7,000 school children died in their classrooms in a single day. Lacking building codes common in the United States, these children died when their poorly constructed schools collapsed during the earthquake. In 2005 an earthquake in Pakistan killed over 17,000 school children, leaving another 50,000 injured or disabled. It is natural and often easy for us to focus intently on our own tragedies; however, the sorrow felt by the parents of 24,000 children who were brutally taken from us and the hundreds of thousands affected in these two incidents should not be missed by the Western world.

We should also be thankful that our efforts have averted untold thousands and perhaps tens of thousands of deaths of American school children through integrated and well-researched building design improvements (Guidance notes, 2009).

Our outlook is a positive one, and we hope that this point comes through to the reader. To illustrate the effectiveness of the concepts outlined in this book, we thought it might be helpful to end our conversation with a few more examples of how tragedy can be overcome. While there are no absolutes when it comes to the prevention of death, these examples all show how proactive approaches can and very often do help us to avert tragedy. These are all success stories that never made the national news because no one died.

Talk Is Cheap

The custodian was walking up the front steps at Alexander II Elementary School in Macon, Georgia. He had a .38 caliber revolver in his back pocket. The butt of the gun was clearly visible, protruding from the pocket as he made his way up the steps to the front door of the school. He was going to use it to kill his wife, who also worked at the school. He was acting irrationally that day. This was exacerbated because he had not taken his insulin. He had somehow become convinced that she was having an affair, and he was determined to shoot her. He was about to enter the school when he heard a loud and clear command voice from behind him ordering him to stop and raise his hands. He stopped, turned, and saw the school district police chief standing next to a police car, pointing a gun at him. He stopped, raised his hands, and surrendered peacefully.

Like many close calls involving acts of violence, this apparently imminent murder was averted because of effective communications at the school district. Indeed, the school district police force had developed a thoughtful and mutually beneficial relationship with the district's custodial services department. That relationship made the district's schools much safer, and developing it cost only a couple of 50-cent cups of coffee.

Dennis Staten and Russell Bentley had developed and then fostered their relationship carefully. This was critical because Staten was the director of custodial services and Bentley was the deputy chief of the school police department. Both men understood how often school custodians can be the first line of defense for the schools they serve. They had regular conversations that created mutual respect, close collaboration, and crystal clear communications. Though the threats they were most concerned about were typically external, the threat in this case had been from one of the department's own personnel. Because of Staten's leadership and communications style, an alert school custodian made a report that a coworker had made concerning statements that foreshadowed the act of violence he was about to carry out. This level of comfort —enough that a line level employee would report this type of information to a supervisor—is a great example of positive relationships and personal initiative in an organization.

Lessons Learned

- Effective communications can be a powerful prevention tool.
- Conversations over a cup of coffee can sometimes be as powerful as a million dollar security system.
- Leaders in organizations can dramatically reduce the risk of violence by establishing open lines of communications.
- Communications and cooperation between security/law enforcement personnel and those they protect can help prevent violence.
- Making people feel comfortable in reporting concerns can save lives.
- Efforts to empower people to take immediate life-saving action should specifically involve instructions to communicate potential danger immediately.

The Star That Didn't Look Right

Officer Levi Rozier was a contentious and dedicated law enforcement officer. The veteran sheriff's deputy had been recruited by the Bibb County School System Police Department because he was deeply respected, intelligent, resourceful, focused on solving problems, and was an excellent communicator. Officer Rozier also demonstrated the attention to detail required of a police officer assigned to the school setting.

While conducting a random surprise metal detection screening of students at Westside High School, Officer Rozier noticed something that caught his eye. He noticed a small object on a male student's keychain. He immediately realized that the symbol was a pentagram.

Because of the intense level of gang activity in the community, school police officers were especially vigilant for any indications that a student was a gang member. This required close attention to numerous warning signs, like the color of a student's shoelaces and various risk-related symbols that could be displayed in an almost infinite fashion on a student's person, clothing, or a notebook. As Officer Rozier carefully but quickly scanned the student's keychain for the small objects containing a blade that officers occasionally found, he had noticed the pentagram.

Understanding that the pentagram could indicate involvement in satanic cult activity, Officer Rozier asked the student to step aside and began a conversation with him. As he asked the student about the pentagram, he became concerned with what he heard. Though the student did not say anything particularly alarming, his responses did not sound quite right for the context of the conversation.

Officer Rozier summoned the members of the district's threat assessment team for assistance. Some years before, the district had pioneered a new concept called multidisciplinary threat assessment. In this approach, a law enforcement officer, school administrator, and a mental health professional work as a team to evaluate situations where threats or behaviors of concern have been noted.

As the team conducted a threat assessment with the student, they became even more concerned. As a result of comments made by the student during the assessment, the student's locker was searched. During the search, a signed suicide pact between the student and his girlfriend was recovered. Both students were committed to residential mental health centers that day. In each student's case, the treating psychologist concluded that the youth was fully committed to committing suicide and that they believed the two students would have done so that afternoon if it were not for the school's intervention.

In Bibb County, the use of multidisciplinary threat assessment helped successfully avert this planned double suicide, a planned middle school bombing, and three planned shooting incidents. Since then, the concept has widely spread to school districts around the nation. This concept has been developed extensively over the last 20 years, and there are now several proven models of threat assessment that schools and other organizations can employ, like the Virginia Model of Student Threat Assessment that we discussed in Chapter Five.

Lessons Learned

- The appropriate use of security technology (in this case a metal detector) combined with the alertness while utilizing the technology helped Officer Rozier spot an item that helped cue him that something was not right.
- Pattern matching helped Officer Rozier detect something was not right about the student with the pentagram.
- The use of multidisciplinary threat assessment helped avert at least two deaths in Bibb County and have since prevented a number of potentially deadly situations.

One Day at a Time

April 16, 2007, was a typical Monday morning for Kristina Anderson, a sophomore at Virginia Tech. Getting up late, Kristina hurriedly jumped into her friend's car for their daily ride to class. Class began at 9:05 A.M., but the two friends did not get there until 9:20. The two toyed with the idea of skipping the class, but in the end they decided to attend anyway.

Being late, Kristina and her friend took a seat on the wall by the door. This placed them in the back left corner of the room as you stood at the front facing the class. The door to the room was to the left, and the windows were to the right, so Kristina sat on the wall next to the hallway.

About 15 minutes after getting to class, Kristina heard the first shots. The sound was sharp and sounded like an axe hitting a piece of wood. As her back was to the wall, she also felt the shock of the shots through the wall. The shots were repetitive, and very quick.

Madame Jocelyne Couture-Nowak, Kristina's professor, went to the door to check on the source of the noise. She looked outside, closed the door quickly, and said, "Call 911!"

The panic in her voice along with her wide-eyed look of terror galvanized some of the students into action. Two of them pushed their desks toward the door in an attempt to barricade the door while Kristina knelt on the floor with her knees under her desk, leaned over her seat, and covered her head with her hands, like she had been taught for earthquake drills.

Before the students could barricade the door, the shooter entered, shot the two students near the door and the professor, and then went toward the windows, shooting her classmates. He reentered the room three times; the third time to shoot himself as police approached.

Kristina ended up being shot twice in the back and once in her toe, most likely the result of a ricochet. She was in intensive care for a week. Her gall bladder was removed, as were parts of her intestines and two-thirds of her left kidney. After a week in the hospital, she was allowed to go home to recover, which involved nearly a month of inactivity as her body healed.

She finished the last two years of her school and graduated on time. But she had periods of hypervigilance, and she felt extreme anxiety the first time she reentered a classroom. Before the attack she felt independent, but afterward she found herself not wanting to be alone, especially at night, when she would cry herself to sleep.

Kristina recalls her therapist teaching her to "empty the trash can," Every session, the therapist had Kristina identify one negative feeling, and they spent the session speaking about that. Taking her recovery one day at a time, Kristina was told that she was having normal reactions to an abnormal situation.

Kristina, who was born in the Ukraine, founded a nonprofit organization dedicated to school safety called the Koshka Foundation for School Safety. The word *koshka* is Russian for "little kitten." Having been the victim of evil directed against her school, Kristina has dedicated her life to protecting others in school and continues to reach out to other survivors (K. Anderson, personal communication, July 20, 2013).

Lessons Learned

- The inability to lock down the classroom resulted in the deaths of the professor as well as most of the students in Kristina's class.
- Prepare in advance by thinking about exit strategies in different scenarios.
- Kristina's seeking and listening to a therapist helped her recover properly.
- Following a traumatic experience, expect the recovery period to be an ongoing daily practice, and to recognize normal reactions to abnormal situations.
- Take your recovery one day at a time.

You Can Do This!

In 2002, a National Armory in Lagos, Nigeria, exploded, resulting in a massive residual sinkhole. Several thousand people were trapped in this sinkhole for seven days. Several hundred people survived by stampeding their way out on the backs and heads of others (Toll in blast, 2002). Many passed out from the climb and the stress of the ordeal, simply giving up and dying.

Sabinah Afuye and her son Turbosun were among the thousands of people trapped in the sinkhole. For days, Sabinah and her son tried climbing out, but it was too steep. Sabinah's health was failing, and she was in need of food, water, and willpower. Turbosun looked at his mother, whose glance told him to forget her and save himself. It was in that moment that he decided defeat was not an option.

Tired, weary, and hungry, he focused inward and began meditating on survival. He placed his mother on his back and began a three-hour climb out of the sinkhole. Every movement was dedicated to staying alive. He finally made it to the top and continued another two miles to the nearest hospital. The death toll rose to over 1,000 people, but the resolve of this young man meant that he and his mother would stay alive.

Sabinah and Turbosun spent the next few months focused on family, faith, and friends to cope with the fact that disaster struck their community.

> Instead of spending my time being angry at the government for causing the blast and doing nothing to help us, I spent my time in church thanking God for sparing my life and my son's life. I don't know how my son managed to climb out of that hole with me, but I'm so happy he had the strength left in his body. I know it was God. (S. Afuye, personal communication, August 16, 2013)

Lessons Learned

- Disasters do not always come from human beings. A sound crisis plan should also cover natural disasters.
- The stampede of panicked individuals trying to escape was among the causes of deaths for over a thousand people in the sinkhole disaster.
- Turbosun's belief in himself allowed him to save his own life and that of his mother.

Moving Forward

In some cases, we will still experience loss in a crisis, but we must continue onward. In 1958, a woman named Maria was the proud wife and mother of six in Guadalajara, Mexico. One day Maria received a phone call from a police officer who informed her that her husband and six children had been in a terrible car accident and were all in critical condition. In that moment, everything changed, and she would be required to focus on holding herself, her family, and her finances together. The first thing Maria did after hanging up the phone was to call the bank where her husband worked. Over the years, she had developed a strong bond with the families of the other employees there as well as the Knights of Columbus at her church. In the past, she and her husband had been regular supporters of these groups through involvement and charitable activities. Now, when she needed it most, the response was overwhelming. She still wept, and she had moments when she didn't know how to continue on, but she had the support of those around her, and she had her faith. She kept faith in herself as much as her family. Maria is another unexpected hero because she did not experience the crisis firsthand; nevertheless, the crisis came to her through her family. In the end, she never gave up on herself or her children, and she never lost sight of their future. As we write this book, she is a proud grandmother who still enjoys life and has the benefit of spending time with her children and their children on a daily basis.

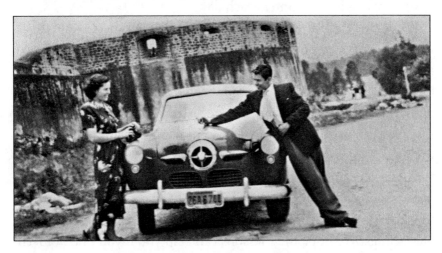

Maria: Like many of the other survivors in this book, Maria Solis survived the loss of her husband and eldest daughter in a terrible car accident through her faith and sense of family. After the wreck, she rented out rooms in her house to earn money to support her family, and now she has four generations of loving and successful children.
Photo: personal collection of the Solis family

Lessons Learned

- Maria's faith and her community allowed her to hold her family together through the loss of a husband and a daughter.
- Seeking help from family, friends, and faith can be useful when recovering from a disaster. In Maria's case, this included working with these groups beforehand to build a sense of community and a safety net.

Life Is Precious

You have seen that there is a wealth of knowledge that can help us survive. The research of the world's leading experts in the fields of psychology and crisis response show us that there are even ways to overcome some of our most primal physical and mental stress responses. We have seen many terrible things in our work, but we write this book with a deep sense of optimism. People now routinely survive many situations that were nearly always fatal a hundred years ago. From disease to mass casualty attacks, we learn more about how to survive deadly encounters each day.

While there will always be tragedy, the stories of success and those who do survive inspire us to rise to the occasion and take the steps needed to survive. Humans are capable of exquisite creations and lofty ideals. We are also capable of terrible acts of depravity that can make you sick to your stomach. Let us only acknowledge the evil that men can do, but focus instead on moving forward with life. The tremendous potential in life is why we seek to protect it.

The people in many of our stories have been family members, friends, and colleagues. These are people we have been truly blessed to meet. They are ordinary people who, under stress, did extraordinary things. We hope their lessons can help you if you find yourself in extraordinary circumstances one day. Remember, you too know amazing people with unique stories of survival. The neighbor who survived a battle with cancer, a coworker who served our nation in combat, and the uncle who saved someone from drowning are all survivors. We can learn a great deal from the people that are all around us. Remember, it's not just about surviving, but living.

Key Points in This Book

- We are much safer today than we were one thousand, one hundred, or even a dozen years ago.
- We now routinely outlive crisis events that were almost always fatal just a few decades ago.
- Survival is not just about staying alive, but being able to move forward mentally as well. Sometimes we need to take things one day at a time.
- You can do this! You can survive a crisis and save others through proper mental preparation.

BIBLIOGRAPHY

Guidance notes on safer school construction. (2009). New York: International Bank for Reconstruction and Development/The World Bank.

Toll in blast at Nigerian armory exceeds 1,000. (2002). *The New York Times.* Retrieved from *http://www.nytimes.com/2002/02/03/world/toll-in-blast-at-nigerian-armory-exceeds-1000.html*

INDEX

ABOUT THE AUTHORS

The coauthors of this book all serve as analysts with Safe Havens International, a nonprofit safety center focused on serving early childcare centers, K–12 schools, institutions of higher learning, and places of worship. Safe Havens analysts have worked in more than two dozen countries and provided assistance to a wide array of organizations including the U.S. Departments of Education, Justice, and Homeland Security. Safe Havens' analysts have authored more than 30 books as well as the U.S. Department of Homeland Security web course IS-360: *Preparing for Mass Casualty Incidents: A Guide for Schools and Houses of Worship*, which was part of the 2013 White House School Safety Initiative. Safe Havens' analysts have assisted in six state-wide school security assessments projects and have assisted clients with school security assessments for more than 6,000 public and nonpublic schools. In addition to their extensive experience as practitioners, they have keynoted hundreds of state, national, and international professional conferences in most of the 50 states as well as Canada, Jamaica, Nigeria, and Vietnam.

Along with their expert witness work, the authors routinely serve as experts for national and international media including *The Wall Street Journal, Education Week, 20/20*, Fox, CNN, NBC, MSNBC, NPR, *The Christian Science Monitor*, Canadian Broadcasting Company, *The Sean Hannity Show*, Al Jazeera America Television, Central China Television, *Time, The Washington Post, The New York Times*, the BBC, and Univision.

Connect with Safe Havens on social media!

Facebook: Facebook.com/SafeHavensIntl
Twitter: @SafeHavensIntl
LinkedIn: Safe Havens International
www.Vimeo.com/SafeHavensIntl
YouTube: *www.youtube.com/SafeHavensIntl*

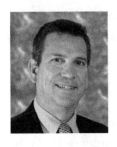

Michael Dorn serves as the Executive Director of Safe Havens International. Michael has published 27 books, and his work has taken him to Central America, Mexico, Canada, Europe, Africa, Asia, and the Middle East. Michael is a graduate of the FBI National Academy 181st session and received a fellowship with the Georgia International Law Enforcement Exchange (GILEE) program, which included travel to Israel for 14 days of orientation and training with the Israel Police, Israel Defense Forces, and the Mossad. Michael had a distinguished 25-year public safety career as a university police lieutenant, school district police chief, school safety specialist for the Georgia Emergency Management Agency—Office of the Governor, and the lead program manager for the Terrorism Division of the Georgia Office of Homeland Security. Michael advised U.S. Attorney General Janet Reno on ways to reduce homicides involving firearms in American schools and worked on the 2013 White House School Safety Initiative. Michael currently serves as a regular guest expert on news networks including CNN, Al Jazeera America, and Fox News.

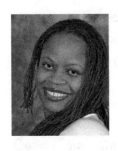

Sonayia N. Shepherd, Ph.D. ("Sony") has authored and coauthored 16 books on school safety and emergency management, including four books for Jane's Information Group. Her unique professional background includes serving as an area school safety coordinator for the nation's largest state school safety center (the School Safety Project in the Georgia Emergency Management Agency—Office of the Governor) as well as the state antiterrorism planner for the Terrorism Division of the Georgia Office of Homeland Security, the state bioterrorism preparedness and emergency response exercise director for the Georgia Department of Public Health, and an incident support specialist for the Centers for Disease Control. An expert in mass casualty event planning, Dr. Shepherd has provided response and

287

recovery support following many school crisis situations and major disasters around the world including Hurricane Katrina, the tsunami in Indonesia, and outbreaks of deadly diseases in Africa and Asia. Dr. Shepherd led the Safe Havens International course authoring team for the 2013 White House School Safety Initiative. She earned her graduate degree in clinical psychology and earned her undergraduate degrees in political science and Spanish. She also holds a Ph.D. in public administration and emergency response policy.

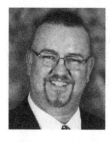

Stephen C. Satterly, Jr. serves as the director of transportation and school safety for an Indiana public school district. He is a certified Indiana school safety specialist and an alumnus of the Indianapolis FBI Citizen's Academy. He has received numerous law enforcement training certifications, including basic certification in the Active Shooter Doctrine and as a Gang Specialist. He has presented at the state and national level and has written for *Campus Safety* magazine, *School Planning and Management* magazine, and *School Transportation News* magazine. He has also served as a research consultant for the 2013 White House School Safety Initiative and has presented at Active Shooter workshops for the U.S. Department of Homeland Security. Steve served as a drill instructor in the U.S. Army, a teacher in a Catholic school, and a middle school principal prior to being selected for his current position.

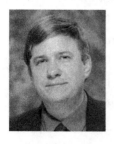

Chris Dorn is an analyst with Safe Havens International. Chris' work in school safety started in 1997 when he was in the seventh grade, and since then his school safety work has taken him across the United States and to Bolivia, Canada, England, France, Holland, Mexico, South Africa, and Vietnam. In addition to serving on the authoring team for the White House Initiative web course, Chris has coauthored six books as well as numerous other publications and is the award-winning executive producer of more than 100 school safety training videos for schools around the world. Organizations that he has trained or that use his training materials include the FBI, TSA, DHS, BATFE, Jane's Consultancy, Israel Police, British intelligence agencies, the International Association of Chief's of Police, the National Association of Pupil Transportation, Vietnam National University, and thousands of law enforcement agencies and school systems in all 50 states and several dozen countries. A graduate of the Georgia Institute of Technology, Chris has a B.A. in international affairs and modern languages with a focus in French and a Certificate of Marketing from Georgia Tech's Scheller College of Business.

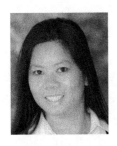

Phuong Nguyen served as the content developer for this project. Her work in bringing together the unique viewpoints of each coauthor to make this book a cohesive work was invaluable. As the director of public information for Safe Havens International, Mrs. Nguyen is a trained and skilled researcher, having completed document preparation for major school safety assessment projects for the Center for Safe Schools funded by Pennsylvania Department of Education, the Hawaii Department of Education, the Maine Department of Education, the Wisconsin Homeland Security Council, the Indiana Department of Education, as well as oversight for all reporting for Safe Havens' school safety assessment projects covering more than 3,000 public, private, charter, independent, and parochial schools. Mrs. Nguyen also served as a research consultant for the web course IS-360: *Preparing for Mass Casualty Incidents: A Guide for Schools and Houses of Worship*, released in June 2013. Mrs. Nguyen holds an M.A. degree in applied linguistics from Vietnam National University and an M.A. in mass communications from Texas Tech University and is presently enrolled in the M.S. dual degree program for Cyber Security/M.B.A. at the University of Maryland University College.

In addition to the authorial team, the following individuals provided their considerable expertise and experience to the development and final review of this book:

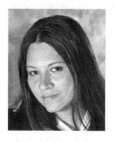

Rachel Wilson serves as the senior photographer for Safe Havens International and is part of the award-winning Safe Havens Video crew. In addition to her work on the photos for this book and her role as producer and videographer for the video supplement, she also worked closely with the authoring team and assisted with content development and review.

Review Team

Rod Ellis is a school district police chief with 26 years of local and state law enforcement experience. Ellis is a published author and certified police instructor. Rod has advanced training in school threat assessment, antiterrorism, emergency planning, and school safety from agencies including the U.S. Departments of Homeland Security and Education, the Georgia Emergency Management Agency, and the Israel Police and security forces.

Les Nichols is the national vice president of child and club safety for Boys & Girls Clubs of America. A passionate and dedicated advocate for children, Nichols is a licensed architect and member of the National Council of Architectural Registration Boards; a board-certified protection professional through the American Society for Industrial Security; a candidate in the Masters of Science in Security Administration program through Southwestern College. For some 20 years, he has worked extensively in all 50 states and on overseas U.S. military installations to improve the safety, security, climate, and culture for youth and those who dedicate themselves to their service.

Gerald Summers is a graduate of the Indiana Law Enforcement Academy and is certified by the Indiana School Safety Specialist Academy (ISSSA) as an advanced school safety specialist. His career includes serving as the coordinator of security and safety for Welborn Baptist Hospital and later the Evansville-Vanderburgh School Corporation in Indiana. He previously served as a police officer for the Evansville Police Department and held similar positions for Bristol Myers Squibb and the Louisville and Nashville Railroad. *Campus Safety* magazine named Summers Campus Safety Director of the Year in the K–12 category in 2012. A graduate of Kennedy Western University with a B.S. in Engineering Safety, Summers served on the Evansville-Vanderburgh School Corporation Board of Trustees for 12 years.

Sue Ann Hartig is a crisis intervention team member certified by the Southwestern Indiana Law Enforcement Academy. She was Executive Director of the Legal Aid Society of Evansville for more than 26 years and also served as the city attorney for the City of Evansville. Hartig was the first female judicial officer appointed in Vanderburgh County. A family and civil mediator, she has taught at University of Evansville, Indiana Vocational Technical College, University of Southern Indiana, and Southwestern Indiana Law Enforcement Academy and currently serves as the volunteer public information officer for the Evansville-Vanderburgh County Emergency Management Agency.

Gregg Champlin is a school emergency planning and natural hazards program specialist for a state-level emergency management agency. Champlin has extensive experience in the field of emergency management and school safety and served as a technical reviewer for *Jane's Safe Schools Planning Guide for All Hazards*, the definitive work on school crisis planning. He has provided advanced training relating to school safety, security, and emergency preparedness for many years, including serving as an instructor for FEMA's Emergency

291

Management Institute for more than 15 years, specializing in school emergency planning and the development of the Introduction to the *Incident Command System for Schools* online course.

Kenneth R. Murray is a police and military trainer whose principles have been adopted by thousands of agencies, nationally and internationally. He serves as an advisor or adjunct instructor for a variety of organizations and conducts extensive training across the United States and Canada. He is the author of *Training at the Speed of Life* and has been regularly published on the topic of simulation training in *Police* magazine, *Law Officer* magazine, *Police Marksman* magazine, and *Police and Security News*.

Dr. Tina S. Brookes is a licensed clinical social worker with more than 20 years of experience as a professional educator. Dr. Brookes has served as a safe school community liaison and a trainer for mental health crisis response. She has also responded to incidents including the tragedies in the Newtown, Connecticut, school shooting; the Aurora, Colorado, movie theater shooting; Hurricane Katrina; and 9/11. She is an approved instructor with the International Critical Incident Stress Foundation and an affiliate faculty member of Resilience Science Institute. Dr. Brookes also regularly presents webinars for organizations like the American Association of Christian Counselors (AACC), where she serves as a board member for the Grief, Crisis and Disaster Network. While assisting with this book, she presented an international webinar for the AACC titled "The Calm Before the Storm: Preparing Schools for Crisis and Disaster."